Women and Girls on the Autism Spectrum

of related interest

Camouflage
The Hidden Lives of Autistic Women
Sarah Bargiela
Illustrated by Sophie Standing
ISBN 978 1 78592 566 5
eISBN 978 1 78592 667 9

Spectrum Women
Walking to the Beat of Autism
Foreword by Lisa Morgan
Edited by Michelle Garnett and Barb Cook
ISBN 978 1 78592 434 7
eISBN 978 1 78450 806 7

Supporting Spectacular Girls
A Practical Guide to Developing Autistic Girls' Wellbeing and Self-Esteem
Helen Clarke
ISBN 978 1 78775 548 2
eISBN 978 1 78775 549 9

Taking Off the Mask
Practical Exercises to Help Understand and Minimise the Effects of Autistic Camouflaging
Dr Hannah Louise Belcher
Foreword by Will Mandy, PhD, DClinPsy
ISBN 978 1 78775 589 5
eISBN 978 1 78775 590 1

Women and Girls on the Autism Spectrum

Understanding Life Experiences from Early Childhood to Old Age

SECOND EDITION

Sarah Hendrickx

With a chapter on eating by Jess Hendrickx

Foreword by Dr Judith Gould

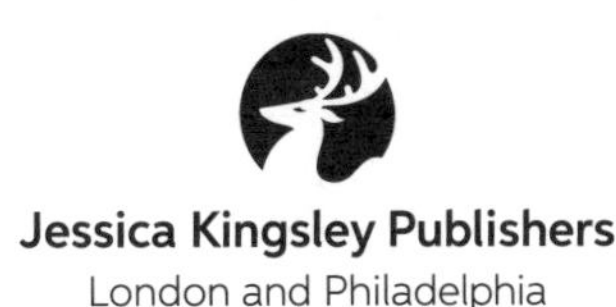

Jessica Kingsley Publishers
London and Philadelphia

First published in Great Britain in 2024 by Jessica Kingsley Publishers
An imprint of John Murray Press

3

A CIP catalogue record for this title is available from the British Library and the Library of Congress

ISBN 978 1 80501 069 2
eISBN 978 1 80501 070 8

Printed and bound in Great Britain by Clays Ltd

Jessica Kingsley Publishers' policy is to use papers that are natural, renewable and recyclable products and made from wood grown in sustainable forests. The logging and manufacturing processes are expected to conform to the environmental regulations of the country of origin.

Jessica Kingsley Publishers
Carmelite House
50 Victoria Embankment
London EC4Y 0DZ

www.jkp.com

John Murray Press
Part of Hodder & Stoughton Ltd
An Hachette Company

For J & J

Sorry about the genes

Contents

Foreword

I was delighted that Sarah Hendrickx had written a second edition of her book *Women and Girls on the Autism Spectrum* and welcomed the opportunity to update my knowledge on this subject.

It is interesting to speculate how much change there has been in the last decade. Diagnosis has improved but still remains a challenge for those women who are adept at camouflaging and masking. It is not the case that we need a new set of diagnostic criteria specifically to address the way in which women and girls present their difficulties; rather it is to understand how females interact with others and how they hide their true selves. Diagnosticians need to be aware of the broader view of how autism is manifested and this book covers the many ways the autistic profile can be recognized. Essentially it is asking the right questions and not taking a narrow view and fitting people into yes/no boxes.

Research in recent years has come closer in understanding the different profiles presented in autism but the question of the male/female ratio of autism prevalence still remains unanswered and is dependant on the selection of participants in various studies. The recent 3:1 ratio is probably an underestimate. The interesting concept of camouflaging and masking has resulted in more research on this subject. The chapter on gender in autism covers these new developments in a clear and informative way.

As in the first edition, the anecdotes and insightful comments presented by autistic women give the book a meaningful dimension with examples of real-life experiences. This, together with the information on updated research, makes the book not only useful but also a fascinating read.

Despite the improvements in diagnosis there are still concerns regarding the use of certain diagnostic tools. Clinicians continue to be rigid in their interpretation of behaviours and depend too heavily on the International Diagnostic Criteria instead of using their clinical judgement and observing the person in different environments. Also, self-report is not merely important but essential as part of the diagnostic process.

Diagnosis in older individuals continues to be problematic when the person has 'hidden' their difficulties by learning the social rules needed to survive in a neurotypical world. This is why it is essential that the diagnosticians have extensive experience to see the autism beneath the observable behaviours. Misdiagnosis has been covered sensitively in the chapter on Health and Wellbeing. The overlap with borderline personality disorder continues to be problematic.

'Collections' of diagnoses is a red flag to the question 'Is this autism?' The benefits of a diagnosis are covered in the chapter on discovery and diagnosis. My experience is that having a diagnosis helps the person come to terms with the way they see the world and subsequently is given the support they need, which in turn helps them to manage their own well-being more effectively.

The section in this chapter on post-diagnostic disclosure gives sound advice on the pros and cons of sharing the diagnosis.

As in the first edition of the book, the chapters discussing the profile through the lifespan from infancy to childhood to later years clearly describe what is needed to know about the positives and pitfalls of being autistic. One major problem addressed is managing uncertainty, which is sensitively discussed and can be the core problem in being autistic. The emphasis on the positive aspects of growing older, such as being comfortable in yourself, is reassuring.

Part III, discussing facets of life, is of particular importance. The chapter on social relationships is excellent, giving very clear and good advice from autistic people themselves with the emphasis on autism being a spectrum. Another important chapter is gender identify and sexuality. Since the first edition of this book there has been much research and discussion around gender identity, which has far reaching implications for autistic females. Sexuality is also a spectrum which shifts and changes through the lifespan.

The chapter on pregnancy and parenting raises many questions often put to those in services providing support. This is essential reading.

In this second edition there is a very informative chapter on eating which is written by Jess Hendrickx, Sarah's daughter. Jess is autistic and therefore has discussed eating difficulties from an autistic perspective. This is much welcomed as this has not sufficiently been dealt with in the past. The chapter is based on Jess's research with autistic women and the mothers of three autistic girls. She emphasizes how much sensory input influences eating difficulties – not just the food. The eating itself is influenced by routines, structures, textures, brands, etc. which are discussed in detail. She then goes on to look specifically at the types of eating disorders seen in autism. The overlap with anorexia nervosa is explained in detail and points out that autism is often missed in a female with eating problems. Losing weight in teenage girls can have many explanations and therefore carrying out a detailed assessment in the light of possible autism is essential.

Health and well-being, particularly mental health, is often not sensitively addressed in autistic individuals. They do not seek medical help or are not listened to. Autistic burnout as a result of the long-term stress of not being understood needs to be addressed by professionals working in the field of mental health and appropriately managed.

The final chapter on living well in a non-autistic world should offer comfort to those on the autistic spectrum as it points out that there is no easy answer but that recognizing and identifying solutions is the way forward.

As in the first edition, this book endorses my clinical experience of working with females on the autistic spectrum and emphasizes the importance of diagnosis at any stage of a person's life. Also, the understanding of neurodiversity has resulted in acceptance of difference in a meaningful way. There have been many positive changes since the first edition of this book. Hopefully these are for the better for all autistic people.

As I did for the first edition I would highly recommend this book for professionals working in the field of autism and for autistic women and girls.

Dr Judith Gould
Consultant Clinical Psychologist
The Lorna Wing Centre for Autism

Acknowledgements

I am indebted to the autistic women and the families of autistic females who took the time to participate by answering my endless questions and helped me in other ways for both this second edition and the first. Some who personally and/or professionally contributed prefer to remain anonymous; others are listed here at their request: Jen Leavesley, Heidi M. Sands, Melanie Peekes, Susan Nairn, Scottish Women's Autism Network (SWAN), Kathleen Comber, Lynda Anderson, Becky Heaver, Kim Richardson, Helen Ellis, Jemimah Pearce, Judith Vaughan, Anna Vaughan, C. Linsky, Emma Dalrymple, Allison Palmer, Claire Robinson, Debbie Allan, Darci, Rose Way, Rachel Sloan, Jade Walker, Makayla Maddison, Anya K. Ustaszewski, Becky Wood and Elle Moore.

I am also very grateful for those – autistic and otherwise – who have been willing to provide their personal and professional experiences. These include Dr Linda Buchan, Steph Jones, Marian Schembari, Dr Catriona Stewart OBE and Florence Neville.

Finally thank you to Jess, my daughter, for contributing a chapter and taking over the empire; and to Keith for typing up the references, for which he has my eternal gratitude because I'm not the right type of autistic for that, and nor is he, but he did it anyway.

Preface

Why?

Welcome to the second edition of this book. Before we go any further, I would like to leave you with an edited version of the original Preface from the first edition, which explains why I wrote it, and I will see you at the other end...

2014

My teenage son was the last in my family to undergo diagnosis for autism, a couple of years after I had received mine. At the appointment, I gave our family history to the psychiatrist carrying out the diagnostic assessment. I included details of my own autism diagnosis and information regarding other members of our family to give some context of an inherited condition. The psychiatrist questioned my diagnosis, asking who had diagnosed me. He asked how I could be autistic because I didn't look like I was autistic, and I was having a two-way conversation with him. I replied that maybe it's because I'm an adult and a woman. He looked at me incredulously and, with obvious contempt, said: 'Are you trying to tell me that being a woman makes a difference?' I replied (sigh) that it did. He shook his head in disbelief. I was furious and sad that the person responsible for my son's (and someone else's daughter's) diagnosis was so ignorant and closed to this possibility. I knew there was nothing I could say. I shut up and hoped that we could just continue with what we had come for. I waited until we had left the room before I cried and exploded with frustration. I wish this was the only occasion where I have had to justify my diagnosis because I don't look autistic enough, but it isn't, and it won't be. And I am not alone in this.

If the gatekeepers of diagnosis and subsequent support are unaware, individuals and families will be powerless to get what they need. The injustice of this makes me unbelievably angry.

This is why I wrote the first edition of this book.

Fast forward ten years...

For the past 17 years – alongside delivering training, conference speaking and running projects in the voluntary sector, education and industry – I have been carrying out non-clinical and clinically supervised autism assessments independently, under contract for part of the UK Ministry of Defence and for a private clinic (Axia-ASD). Over this time, the demographic of those who have sought autism assessment has entirely changed. Initially, the people who came were all male, often 'encouraged' by a female partner who had deemed their behaviour as possibly autistic, and then a trickle of females began to come along. As time has gone by, my clients are around 99 per cent female. What changed? Awareness, that's what. I am humbled and honoured that the first edition of this book has been cited by many women as one of the catalysts for them seeking verification of their suspicions about being autistic.

With the help of the females in the first edition of this book who shared their voices and their stories – and along with all other autistic females who speak, write, make videos and advocate – a huge number of autistic women have felt the relief of the 'that's me' lightbulb moment that so many of them describe. They have felt the liberation of knowing they were not broken and that they are not alone.

For the first edition I carried out a literature review of all academic papers about gender-related autism and found a shockingly small number of fewer than 20 papers. That number has grown over the past seven years to hundreds, if not thousands, and so it's time that things are brought up to date. We know more about masking, parenting, food, menopause, interests and sensory differences for females than we did when I began, so those topics too are covered more fully in this second edition. I have found a new group of autistic women willing to answer my new questions and share their experiences on a broader range of topics, and have used the expertise of my (autistic) daughter, Jess, for a whole new chapter on eating. It's going to be very exciting.

If you bought the first edition and have now purchased this second edition, then I thank you and hope that the new content adds to your knowledge and validation. If you are new to this book, I thank you also, and welcome you to a world of discovery about the private and public worlds of as many autistic women as I could find along with a load of other stuff that 'official' academic people have written about us.

INTRODUCTION

Since the beginning of our modern-day understanding of autism, shared by the likes of Kanner and Asperger, the consensus has been that there are substantially more males with the condition than there are females. I frequently discussed this with people attending the training courses that I delivered, and the overwhelming opinion was that there are more autistic males than females and 'that's just the way it is'. The professionals attending these courses held this belief because they stated they had more male autistic clients/pupils/patients than female, therefore it must be true. Others expressed surprise that women could be autistic at all, because they had never knowingly met an autistic woman.

Increasingly, the questioning of the origin of this 'fact', aided by the increased profile of autistic females in research, the media and in awareness events, has given rise to a new understanding: that is, there are plenty of autistic women, but we just hide it better (but often at great cost). We make sense of it differently or present it in a way that slips under the radar of those looking for classic (male) indicators derived from the (almost) exclusively male research, or at least research that did not until very recently differentiate according to gender.

We still have a way to go to educate important and influential people who are necessary for the support and care of autistic females as to the real picture, but we are getting there. The prevalence of awareness sessions, conferences and projects all focused on so-called 'female autism' demonstrate this change in perception of what autism might look like. These events and initiatives did not exist when I wrote the first edition of this book. This is real progress, although for those on the front line looking for accurate assessment, help and understanding, it may not always feel that way.

I am one of those autistic women who has hidden it extremely well, to the point that I couldn't even see it myself. I say 'hidden', although this was not a conscious ploy – more a subconscious response to a lifelong understanding that the 'real me' was not usually particularly welcome or approved of. I have wanted to get by with the minimum of conflict and I prefer not to be visible, for the wrong reasons. Therefore, I have used my rather capable brain to work out how to do that with relative success (despite considerable harm to myself mentally and physically) and through constant rehearsal, monitoring, observation, mimicry and a whole host of other exhausting strategic measures. Even then, the flash of puzzled confusion across someone's face at what I have just said or done doesn't appear to diminish with age or effort. This is what is now referred to as 'camouflaging'.

I was diagnosed as autistic at the age of 43 years. At this point in my life I had been working exclusively in the field of autism for five years, both as an employee and as a self-employed person running my own autism and neurodiversity training, assessment and coaching organization, Hendrickx Associates (now run by my autistic daughter, Jess).[1] I had completed a master's degree in autism, written five books on autism, spoken at many conferences, trained several thousand practitioners in autism and worked with several hundred autistic individuals. It seems ludicrous even to me that someone so immersed in both the theory and practice of autism could not 'spot' it in herself.

The reason that it took me so long to do so was that I was guilty of doing exactly the same thing that everyone else had been doing to autistic women for all those years: I was comparing myself with the male presentation, and it didn't fit. Specifically, I was using my autistic partner, Keith, as my control sample. In fact, I was so

1 www. hendrickxautism.com

convinced of my somewhat neurotypical (NT) status that Keith and I wrote a book about our Asperger syndrome (AS)/NT relationship (Hendrickx and Newton, 2007) and the differences between our neurology, and how clever I was at being able to understand his despite not sharing it.

Over time, I realized that we were actually very similar in numerous ways and that I just 'got' him in a way that most people had struggled to do, and that equally, with him I was able to exist in my natural state without fear. I learned how incredibly logical, routine orientated and systematic I am, but with none of the interest in technical things he has. My fascination is people and how they operate – most typically articulated by a frown and 'Why do they do that?', although I don't know why I persist in asking Keith as he has less of a clue than I do. I realized that I have always struggled enormously socially yet have persisted in adopting an utterly exhausting, extroverted persona to socialize anyway at great mental cost to myself because I am supposed to, whereas he will just say 'no' and avoid any discomfort.

For several years, my analytical, self-obsessed nature was having a ball trying to work out the paradox of how Keith and I could be so different and yet so similar. The realization and the answer came slowly and steadily every time I met an autistic woman through my work as an autism specialist and coach. I would work with autistic women professionally – even assessing them for autism – and, on hearing their life stories and their way of being, I was frequently shocked by the similarity between their lives and my own. Numerous failed relationships and failed jobs; many jettisoned, short-lived projects where a previously all-encompassing interest disappeared overnight; anxiety and 'madness' (to quote numerous people in my own life) – it was all so familiar. I could see precisely how these things fitted the diagnostic criteria for them, and I was then able to begin applying that understanding to myself. After a few more years of data-gathering and self-analysis, I went for a diagnosis and my suspicions were unreservedly confirmed. In the intervening years between then and now, the majority of my wider family over at least four generations have one by one been diagnosed (or self-identified) with a range of neurodiverse conditions and/or other features often associated with autism (including autism, dyslexia, attention deficit hyperactivity disorder (ADHD), tic disorders, Ehlers–Danlos syndrome, transgender, non-binary gender identity), so it seems I may not have been alone here.

Ironically, I felt that working in the field of autism made it harder for me to 'come out' – there were only a very small number of openly autistic speakers and professionals at that time, so my role models were few. I had been surrounded by it and studied it and yet hadn't realized I was it myself. My outward presentation is extremely well constructed. My lifelong special interest in studying people has both served me well but hidden the truth: that I am struggling and exhausted most of the time. The aim of this life's work of mine has been to learn how to be invisible and never appear less than 100 per cent perfect and capable. The prospect of disclosure and admitting to actually being different – and (in my eyes) less than the perfectly acceptable person I have always striven to be – was a huge personal dilemma. I have never considered autistic people as inadequate, but my own logic results in me applying these ridiculous standards to myself. I am also fully aware of the level of discrimination that autistic people experience and felt that professional disclosure could affect people's willingness to work with me – and I had bills to pay. So, at the same time as supporting recently diagnosed individuals on a professional basis, I was coming to terms with my own diagnosis and what this meant for me psychologically and practically.

It took me three years following my diagnosis to tell anyone beyond my immediate family. The response professionally was overwhelmingly positive, but the dichotomy of being both authentic and visible, and striving to be invisible, remains. Fifty-five years (and counting) of trying to perfect the 'normal' persona is difficult to drop, although increasingly – with grateful thanks to menopause, recurring autistic burnout and ageing – my need and energy to maintain the pretence are just about gone.

My personal journey as an autistic person continues every minute of every day. The knowing is just the start; the understanding and the living as an autistic in a non-autistic world never ends. Almost every day I learn new things that make sense of decades of confusion. Knowledge of the way life is experienced by women on the autism spectrum is relatively new and not yet fully understood, except by the women themselves. The women have been living this way forever but have only recently started to learn the vocabulary to explain it.

This book is not a definitive picture of life for all autistic women; it is a small sample from a large and varied community designed to broaden understanding and, I hope, offer support. I have assessed over a thousand autistic women, and what I have presented here are experiences common to many of them along with as many research papers as I could read and digest, although there are so many now that I had to force myself reluctantly to stop through lack of time after reading 200 or so – such a different picture from when I wrote the first edition of this book. It is the best I could do, and I hope it's okay. The inclusion of some of my own experiences is not intended to appear self-indulgent; I just wanted to include as many voices as I could. My experience is no more representative than anyone else's. We're all different, yet all the same.

I hope that through this work professionals will consider new indicators to look for and will ask different questions when assessing females; that practitioners will see past the personas and not disbelieve; and that women who suspect they are autistic will find solidarity, shared experiences and the courage to seek diagnosis if that is what they need. Many highly esteemed professionals and autistic individuals are recognizing the idea that gender might matter when considering the diagnosis, profile and support of autism in females. I hope to share their work and add a little of my own to the conversation.

This book does not seek to detract from a more traditionally reported experience of autism, but rather to present a missing piece of the partial picture that has been in the public domain for many years. Almost all of the initial research into autism was carried out on boys, and their profile was deemed to be the default, so it is not surprising that girls and others who identify with a different presentation never got much of a look-in. Gender was never considered an issue, but it might be for some at least. The girls have been missed because no one took the time to look for them. And the girls need to know who they are.

For information

This book assumes the reader has some basic knowledge of autism spectrum disorder (ASD) and its characteristics. I have not gone into detail regarding standard theoretical concepts and behaviours, beyond those that are specifically relevant to females and the literature. There are many other superb publications by well-respected authors who have done this. Characteristics presented may be indicative of autism, but may also, when considered in isolation, be caused by something else. The inclusion of characteristics does not imply that autism is the only explanation for them. This book does not give the reader the knowledge or experience to make a diagnosis of autism and it should be used in conjunction with expert advice and assessment.

I have used the terms 'female', 'girl' and 'woman' for ease of explanation given the focus of the book, but no intention is intended to exclude non-binary, male, trans or others who identify with this profile. I have always been clear that the concept of 'female autism' is currently misleading, undefined and not gender specific, and that this is simply a broader view of how autism may present in any human.

The anonymous verbatim quotes used throughout the book come from a group of autistic women and parents of autistic girls who agreed to contribute. They all contributed via emailed questionnaires and personal conversations during 2014 (first edition) and 2022/23 (second edition) on a variety of topics as covered in the chapters. In total, over 45 females shared their experiences. Some contributed more and/or different information than others due to age and specific life experiences (e.g. whether they were parents or had experience of employment). The contributors were mainly from the UK and USA. Ages ranged from 5 to 76 years. Most were white with a very small number from ethnic backgrounds. All of their words are indented from the margin. Any first-person experiences that are not indented from the margin are my words, about my life.

The term 'autism spectrum disorder' (ASD) is used throughout to reflect the *Diagnostic and Statistical Manual of Mental Disorders Fifth Edition* (DSM-5, American Psychiatric Association, 2013) specification and to encompass all forms of autism. 'Neurotypical' (NT) is used as a term to describe those not on the autism spectrum and with a neurologically typical profile. It is a standard term used for ease, not to homogenize any group. Within quoted contributor and reference responses, terms such as 'Aspie', 'Asperger syndrome' and 'high-functioning autism' are used. These are the contributors' own words. I have not by choice used the terms 'high-functioning', 'low-functioning', 'mild' and 'severe' to describe an autistic person, as they are misleading, unhelpful and usually wrongly aligned to developmental/intellectual ability. If I have used any of these terms in this book, they will either be qualified and specific in definition, or will be other people's terminology that I am quoting or referencing. The same principle applies to terms such as 'deficit', 'wrong', 'amiss' or 'abnormal' – this is the researchers' or participants' terminology that is being reproduced, not my own perspective. If some quotes appear negative, this is to provide a broad view of different perspectives of autism along with the thoughts and terminology of those affected, rather than any personal opinion of my own. My aim is to show the breadth of experience of living on the autism spectrum in an otherwise non-autistic world.

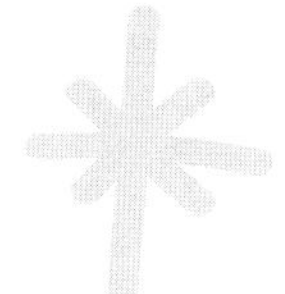

Part I

THEORY AND DIAGNOSIS

Chapter 1

GENDER IN AUTISM

Background to autism in females

Autism spectrum disorder (ASD) is a broad, complex and still, apparently, relatively unfathomable condition, although knowledge and understanding about it is constantly expanding. Data gathered by the Centers for Disease Control and Prevention in the US in 2018 suggests that 1 in 44 people have ASD, but the actual number is likely to be much higher due to the underdiagnosis of older people and females.

We are learning that autism is a more diverse disorder than was originally described by Dr Kanner more than 70 years ago. Yet despite all the recent breakthroughs in research, we still can't explain exactly what it is; we're not even close. And then there is the matter of gender in autism as well. Research that investigates and differentiates the male and female profile, presentation and experience of autism has been extremely scarce up until the past five to ten years, perpetuating by default the view that autism is a significantly male-dominated condition, or, alternatively, that gender is simply not something worthy of consideration.

Although the development of the original diagnostic profile was based almost entirely on a male phenotype (Kopp and Gillberg, 1992), it is important to note that mention was made of the possibility of autistic females by both Leo Kanner and Hans Asperger in the 1940s. Kanner (1943) had noted that one girl did not understand games and pretended to be a dog, walking on all fours and making dog noises, and Asperger wondered whether autism may not present itself in girls until puberty, given that he had not encountered any females in his studies of younger children.

Due to the paucity of diagnosed autistic women until recent years, it has been difficult to find sufficient numbers of age- and developmentally matched females to participate in research that might show significant findings (Mandy *et al.*, 2012). Put simply, if girls are not getting diagnosed because the criteria do not pick them up (because they weren't considered in the creation of the criteria), there will be fewer women diagnosed and able to be included in research samples; research will therefore draw conclusions from smaller samples of the females who do match the male criteria... and on it goes...

Many esteemed individuals working in the autism field have commented, and considered for several years, that what is now being referred to as 'female ASD' is worthy of differentiation from the standard profile; they include Tony Attwood, Simon Baron-Cohen, Svenny Kopp, Francesca Happé, Dr William Mandy, Lorna Wing and Judith Gould.

It is also the case that the autobiographical and anecdotal published works on autism have had a plethora of autistic women as authors for many years: Temple Grandin, Laura James, Rudy Simone, Yenn Purkis, Marian Schembari, Purple Ella and Robyn Steward, to name but a few. It seems that the women themselves have the words and the desire to speak out about their lives, but that research is only just beginning to catch up and concede that they exist and are worthy of individual attention.

We also have to consider that the tools used for identifying autism may have a male gender bias and therefore are not 'picking up' female autism if it has a distinctly separate neurological or behavioural quality. ASDs are currently diagnosed behaviourally and observationally, therefore despite any potential similarities or differences on a cognitive or neurodevelopmental level, it may simply be that females present their autism differently through behaviours that are not included in the current diagnostic criteria (Kopp and Gillberg, 1992) or are masking them with great success. If this is the case, it is likely that clinicians making diagnoses need to view the current criteria more broadly to ensure that female behaviour is considered.

Over the years, there have been many differing opinions on the male:female ratios of autism prevalence. A large-scale review, which examined 54 studies – with a total of almost 14 million participants, 53,712 of whom had autism diagnoses – found that the male:female ratio for autism is close to 3:1 and that there seems to be a gender bias, resulting in girls who meet the diagnostic criteria not being given a clinical diagnosis (Loomes *et al.*, 2017). It has also been found elsewhere that girls were significantly less likely to receive an autism spectrum diagnosis than boys, even when their symptoms were equally severe (Russell, Steer and Golding, 2011), perhaps due to gender expectations and stereotyping by parents and professionals. Theories such as the 'extreme male brain theory' (Baron-Cohen, 2002) may also have contributed to the popular view of autism as a 'male' condition, which may influence professionals in their consideration of autism as a likely diagnosis for a female. All of these factors may suggest that the 3:1 reported ratio continues to under estimate the true number of autistic females.

Nature of the difference between genders

There are varying perspectives as to the nature of male–female autism (Lai *et al.*, 2011), but until very recently almost every single one of these comparative studies has been carried out on children rather than adults, and so is far from the complete picture. One is that male and female autism may differ on a neurological and/or cognitive level (Carter *et al.*, 2007). Another suggests that perhaps there are fewer autistic females because they are somehow protected against developing the condition (Volkmar, Szatmari and Sparrow, 1993; Jacquemont *et al.*, 2014), which may also explain why many neurodevelopmental conditions appear to affect more males than females (Zahn-Waxler, Shirtcliff and Marceau, 2008). While sex differences in autism have been largely ignored (Bölte *et al.*, 2011), there is a small amount of work that has considered neurological perspectives of differences in brain development and functioning as potential factors in explaining male and female autism. Lai *et al.* (2013) found that aspects of brain neuro-anatomy are sex dependent. Furthermore, this study also found minimal overlap between the neuro-anatomical features of males and autistic females, suggesting that males and autistic females may actually be neurally and cognitively distinct. Craig *et al.* (2007) found differences in the density of grey and white matter in areas of the brain linked to social behaviour deficit in autistic women compared to neurotypical women. The autistic women's brains were similar to those of autistic males.

One theory is that autistic females are somehow 'more impaired' than autistic males and that perhaps the neural or cognitive 'damage' that has to occur in order for a female to be autistic needs to be greater than for a male. One study found that girls with 'high-functioning' autism who attended a clinic were 'more neuro-cognitively affected' (Nyden, Hjelmquist and Gilberg, 2000, p.185) than boys with the same diagnosis attending the same clinic. The girls were seen to have more 'extensive deficits' in theory of mind and executive functioning than the boys. The study suggests that girls attending the clinic may be in greater need of support than the boys (Nyden *et al.*, 2000). Volkmar *et al.* (1993) found that, in IQ testing, larger numbers of autistic females were at the lower end of the IQ scale and had intellectual disabilities than males, which appears to support the suggestion above that, in general, autism needs to be 'worse' for it to manifest in women, with fewer women appearing in the intellectually typical category of autism. Other work has similar findings (Wing, 1981; Lord, Schopler and Revicki, 1982; Tsai and Beisler, 1983) although due to the age of these papers, these observations will not have taken into account the tendency for intellectually able autistic females to mask, or even the presence of an autistic profile without intellectual disability (formally categorized as Asperger syndrome, which did not enter diagnostic manuals until 1994) which may have hidden their true numbers.

Professor Simon Baron-Cohen and other researchers from the Autism Research Centre in Cambridge, UK, have been studying prenatal androgen exposure and other neurobiologically occurring chemicals in autistic children. Several studies focus on the 'extreme male brain theory' of autism developed by Baron-Cohen (2002) and how this manifests in women. The concept of masculinized behaviour in autistic females is one of the more researched areas in gender difference, which has had mixed reactions from the autism community – some find it too binary in nature in describing all behaviour as either masculine or feminine. According to the prenatal testosterone theory of autism (Ingudomnukul *et al.*, 2007; Auyeung *et al.*, 2009), autism may be caused by elevated foetal testosterone levels and prenatal androgen exposure. These levels are correlated both positively and inversely with a number of autistic characteristics, including eye contact, vocabulary and social relationships. Further research revisiting these ideas (Bejerot *et al.*, 2012) confirms that testosterone levels in autistic women were higher than control samples and that these women displayed more 'masculinized' characteristics. It also found that autistic men presented more 'feminized' characteristics, indicating that rather than autistic women being more masculinized *per se*, both genders may be more androgynous and represent a 'gender defiant disorder' (Bejerot *et al.*, 2012, p.9). They go on to suggest that 'gender incoherence in autistic individuals is to be expected and should be regarded as one reflection of the wide autism phenotype' (p.9). This may be reflected in the atypical gender identity and sexuality profiles often seen in autistic females, which will be discussed later in this book as will the notion that autistic females can present a profile – physically, cognitively and/or behaviourally – less stereotypically feminized than that of neurotypical (NT) females.

Another study looked specifically at one element of behaviour and compared response inhibition in males and autistic females (Lemon *et al.*, 2011). Individuals were asked to respond to a light being switched on by pressing a button as quickly as possible. The study found that autistic females were significantly slower to *stop* responding (i.e. to inhibit their responses) than either autistic males or NT males and females. Autistic males did not show any difference in response inhibition times to NT males and females. This study only focuses on one small area of behaviour but may suggest that autistic females have a different neurobehavioural profile to autistic males. The consequences of impaired inhibitory control include impulsiveness, risk-taking and general executive dysfunction, including planning and decision-making. This may also impact on other social difficulties, such as appropriate behavioural responses, particularly when under stress (Lemon *et al.*, 2011).

Carter *et al.* (2007) looked at sex differences in autistic toddlers and found that girls scored more highly in visual reception than boys, while boys scored more highly in language, motor and social competence than girls. They report statistically significant cognitive and development profile differences between girls and autistic boys aged one to three years. A study of a similar age group (Hartley and Sikora, 2009) found many parallels in the male and female profile, but some 'subtle but potentially important differences between the male and female ASD phenotype' (p.179). Boys showed more repetitive, restricted behaviours than girls, and girls showed more communication deficits, sleep problems and anxiety. Girls had more 'emotional problems' (Mandy *et al.*, 2012, p.1310) and better fine motor skills, and as with other studies (Wilson *et al.*, 2016), restricted, repetitive behaviour was seen less in girls than in boys.

Bölte *et al.* (2011) found that executive functioning was scored more highly in autistic girls, and attention to detail was scored more highly in autistic boys. This may add weight to the suggestion that autistic boys show more stereotypical ritualized behaviours than autistic girls (Carter *et al.*, 2007). Kopp and Gillberg's (2011) later work found that the following behaviours were much more typical of autistic girls than boys: 'avoids demands', 'very determined', 'careless with physical appearance' and 'interacts mostly with younger children' (pp.2881–2882).

Camouflaging/masking

> People praise us for what we are capable of and what we have achieved thanks to our performance... but no one stops to consider the toll it takes on us (Higgins *et al.* 2021, p.2361)

> Masking is a tool that should be used to get things, nothing more nothing less. Like with anything in life, overdoing it leads to problems. With masking there can be quite serious burnout, forgetting who you are, constant anxiety from fear of slipping and being exposed. (Mantzalas *et al.*, 2022, p.58)

Camouflaging is defined as 'the use of conscious or unconscious strategies, which may be explicitly learned or implicitly developed, to minimize the appearance of autistic characteristics during a social setting' (Hull, Petrides and Mandy, 2020, p.309). Masking, compensation and assimilation are all part of the same process by which autistic people attempt to change their behaviours, having become aware that their natural selves are not perceived as socially acceptable. A number of women describe themselves as 'chameleons' in the way that they adapt, adopt personas, mimic and become invisible in social settings as a way not to be visible for the wrong reasons and attract negative attention.

Lai *et al.* (2011) found that on comparing boys and autistic girls, both were 'equally autistic' (p.5) as children, but that as adults the females showed fewer social communication difficulties, suggesting that they may have learned compensatory strategies and may be more motivated to do so throughout their lives in order to appear more 'socially typical' (p.6). The men in this study had not followed the same trajectory into adulthood. This behaviour of 'acting as if neurologically typical' (Lai *et al.*, 2019) is termed 'camouflaging' or 'masking'. It is suggested that autistic women are able to apply the systematic nature of their autistic brain (Baron-Cohen, 2002) to the study and replication of people skills in order to imitate and participate socially. However, the mechanical (rather than intuitive) basis of these strategies means that at times of stress, in unexpected situations or after a period of time, it may be impossible for them to be maintained (Lai *et al.*, 2011). For some women this can mean that they present a very capable front that cannot be maintained beyond certain limits, after which it collapses (and sometimes so does she).

Later diagnosis amongst females may be explained by females

with high autistic traits being less likely to show clinically significant features due to a superior ability to compensate (Livingston and Happé, 2017). It has also been suggested that autistic women are better at masking their autistic features due to better self-awareness and self-referential abilities (Attwood, 2007; Lai *et al.*, 2011). This increased ability would support women's reported improved understanding of what is required socially and how to meet these expectations. Dr Linda Buchan, clinical psychologist and Director of Axia-ASD clinic, reports how a desire to fit in and join groups can lead to more disadvantageous masking in those of lower economic backgrounds. She suggests that working-class autistic women can get more easily sucked into crime and drugs via this behaviour which, combined with a difficulty in seeing hidden agendas, can lead to serious outcomes. Middle-class autistic women, she argues, may be more likely to join safer groups through masking.

> I honed something of a persona which was kind of bubbly and vivacious, and maybe a bit dim, because I had nothing to say other than adult novels. So, I cultivated an image, I suppose, that I brought out to social situations as my partner's girlfriend, that was not 'me'. (Bargiela, Steward and Mandy, 2016, p.3287)

Comments on females' ability to appear socially typical and mask their autistic behaviours occur in the literature time and time again (Attwood, 2007; Gould and Ashton-Smith, 2011; Lai *et al.*, 2011), but it is only very recently that professionals in the field have attempted to formalize this to improve the situation through the development of camouflaging screening tests and studying the lived experiences of autistic women to uncover their compensation strategies and their impacts.

Autistic women of colour

There was a time when locally – I live in a fairly large city – and I could go to events that were related to autism and I kind of played

> *this game called Spot the Person of Color; it was a game I played with myself. Because typically there were almost no people that looked like me or that seemed to be a person of color.*
>
> Morénike Giwa Onaiwu, Autism Women's Network (Rozsa, 2017)

If being female makes it difficult enough to be recognized as autistic, being a female of colour makes it almost impossible. The US Centers for Disease Control and Prevention hold no information on the race or ethnicity of autistic adults but states that 'whites are 30% more likely to receive an autism diagnosis than blacks and are 50% more likely to receive a diagnosis than Hispanics' (Full Spectrum Child Care, 2020); and in an analysis of 408 peer-reviewed articles on autism treatments, only 17.9 per cent of them mentioned the ethnicity or race of the participants (West *et al.*, 2016) and of those that did so, 63.5 per cent of the participants were white.

Some black autistic women are sharing their experiences of the intersection between autism and race. Catina Burkett (2020) describes how at work she is subjected to stereotypes within both the white and the black community of how she should behave as a black woman as well as an autistic woman, and appears to fail to meet both in the eyes of others due to her inability to 'code switch' and change her tone of voice and mannerisms to fit in with different people regardless of their ethnicity. Morénike Giwa Onaiwu (Rozsa, 2017) also talks about how her race has impacted how she has been treated as an autistic woman:

> I believe that my experiences as an autistic person have definitely been affected by my gender and race. Many characteristics that I possess that are clearly autistic were instead attributed to my race or gender. As a result, not only was I deprived of supports that would have been helpful, I was misunderstood and also, at times, mistreated.

Morénike goes on to give an example of how her autistic features have been wrongly attributed to her race and culture:

> So eye contact is something that I've never been good at, it's variable. Sometimes I can do it, sometimes I can't, and I'm African American; I'm also of African descent – my parents are African immigrants. I think my teachers would say, 'Oh well she's, you know, West African. They don't look people in the eye because that's considered to be rude'. (Rozsa, 2017)

In the United States, getting an autism diagnosis comes later if you are non-white and/or have an accompanying intellectual disability (Wiggins *et al.*, 2019), meaning that 'autistic black girls are effectively invisible in the current scientific literature' (Diemer, Gerstein and Regester, 2022). The authors suggest that screening all children for autism would improve the chances of those from all racial/ethnic backgrounds having an equal chance of being diagnosed, which would also provide a more representative sample for future research.

Chapter 2

DISCOVERY AND DIAGNOSIS

Considering autism

There is a huge range in the ages of individuals and the circumstances in which they or their families first considered that autism might be part of their picture. For most adult women, autism could not have been offered as a possible explanation for their differences due to the relatively recent understanding of autism in females. Younger girls have had this opportunity much earlier in their lives, the commonly mentioned 'lightbulb' moment coming to a parent rather than the individual themselves.

> Age four, after reading about how girls manifest their symptoms differently to boys, I just knew. (Parent)

> [...] Random suggestion over lunch with a child psychologist doing a garden tour on the other side of the country. She had just completed a piece of research that matched my daughter's struggles in life after having relationships in adult life that left her vulnerable to violence and financial exploitation. (Parent)

> I had always felt 'different' and excluded by others and wanted to know why. A friend was going for an assessment, and I realized I didn't know as much about autism as I thought I did. I read a personal account of having Asperger's by a woman on

> the Internet and it made me cry with recognition – I knew I had to explore the possibility so that I could at least rule it in or out.

> My son was diagnosed and as I sat in conferences regarding ASD [autism spectrum disorder], I sat there going tick, tick to myself [...] therefore got diagnosis.

For some, autism wasn't on their radar, but a definite sense of 'difference' certainly was – and sometimes from a very young age.

> When I started school, I noticed everyone else was different to me, but after a while I realized I was the one who was different and not them.

> We were trying to figure out why all schools kicked her out. Why she had no friends. Why she couldn't keep a job. (Parent)

Both adult women and parents of girls talk about feeling doubt about their suspicions, due to not entirely meeting the traditional (male) profile that has proliferated, and not being believed when sharing their thoughts about possible autism with others. In the case of some individuals, their own lack of general understanding about the spectrum of autism caused them to react negatively when it was suggested as a cause of their child's or their own presentation.

> My mother said, 'Do you think she's autistic?' when she was three weeks old. I was furious. She was a very difficult baby for many reasons, and it was obvious that she was 'different' from the beginning. I have some severely autistic relatives and I didn't know that there were degrees of autism. I ruled it out because I thought she was much too clever to be 'autistic' [...] It was only when the nursery told me to look up Asperger syndrome on the Internet that I finally realized what we were dealing with. (Parent)

> I was 26 when I first started to think I could be autistic. I saw

> something on TV about a girl who had Asperger's [...] I could relate to everything she said. Up until that moment, I thought Asperger's was only found in males.

There are many fascinating paths that have led adult women to the realization that autism may be an explanation for the experiences that they have had. Often women had spent many decades searching for an answer that fitted, frequently exploring and discarding other explanations along the way. Mariam Schembari, autistic author of *A Little Less Broken* (forthcoming) explains:

> I didn't [think that I was autistic]. It literally never crossed my mind. I thought autism was a young boy obsessed with trains and flapping his hands... What finally triggered the connection for me was watching a friend's Instagram video. Her son had recently been diagnosed, which led to her diagnosis. As she talked, something clicked in me. She and I were so similar, and a lot of the traits she mentioned...made me immediately Google, 'Am I autistic?' I took a short test, which led me down the rabbit hole of information on how it presents so differently in marginalized genders. I had no idea. (Schembari, pers. comm., 2023)

> I had always identified as a Highly Sensitive Person and put it all down to my personality type (INFJ [Myers–Briggs personality type 'introverted, intuitive, feeling and judging']). I have spent my life studying human beings because it's as though I didn't quite get the memo in how to behave.

> My initial response (to the realization of possible autism) was that of mind-blowing explosions in my head which lasted about a year. I was very much in shock I think but over the moon that I'd recognized my struggles were not psychological but neurological, and finding a community of other like-minded people who saw life as I do. There was a massive grief process that ran alongside it too as I updated my entire self-concept and reviewed my history through a new perspective.

Accessing diagnosis

Increasing the autism education of professionals and clinicians working at all points along the diagnostic and support pathway has to be the number one priority to ensure accurate assessment. In many cases, sadly, this is the stumbling block to appropriate support since referrals and evidence may be required from these people to allow a positive autism diagnosis to be given. A study of mental health professionals in one region of England found that 79 per cent of people rated their own knowledge of autism as 'limited' or 'fair', and 59 per cent said that they had not received any autism training within the past two years. The same study asked autistic service users for their perceptions of mental health services and found that only 17 per cent felt that staff understood their needs relating to having autism and only 23 per cent were satisfied with the mental health support they received (Impact Initiatives, Asperger's Voice Self-Advocacy Group and West Sussex Asperger Awareness Group, 2013). Even those who had a positive experience in the end often appeared to have overcome an obstacle course to get there.

> [...] A wonderful psychiatric paediatrician at the local hospital [...] He was the first person who had ever treated us like 'good' parents, who listened to us and to my daughter and was kind, respectful and incredibly helpful. This followed years of horrible professionals giving us misleading diagnoses and making us feel like we were dreadful people. (Parent)

When they seek diagnosis, frightening comments of professional ignorance are reported:

> The neurobehavioural team [autism diagnostic service] only takes referrals from consultant psychiatrists in the mental health team, and the mental health team didn't understand autism so wouldn't refer me as they thought that autism was only so-called 'classic' autism and didn't understand that it was a spectrum.

> [UK state diagnostic service] were a disaster – openly admitted they didn't understand autistic girls. (Eaton, 2012, p.11)

> The psychologist told me she didn't know girls could get it [autism]. (Eaton, 2012, p.11)

> The GP said that autism doesn't exist and that it is all down to bad parenting. He told me I should spend more time with my kids. He was even willing to put this down in writing. (Parent – this event happened in 2022, which shows that progress is still to be made.)

> Mr X (the clinician) began talking about how if a person/child behaves differently in different environments then they cannot be autistic. I told him I did not agree with this, and it is not my own personal experience of autism. I discussed masking. His response was 'masking is just a part of life for everyone; people do not understand this'... I also told him that when I spoke to my GP about this referral...she mentioned autism. Mr X's response was 'your GP doesn't understand autism'. (Parent)

> I'll always remember my special needs teacher saying I'm too poor at maths to be autistic. (Bargiela *et al.*, 2016, p. 3286)

> We moved to The Netherlands two years later and she was eventually diagnosed with Asperger syndrome there at the local children's hospital. We thought the Dutch were very liberal and forward thinking but they, to our horror, suggested that A would be better off institutionalized! (Parent)

> [The diagnosis] only took a couple of hours looking at school records and history. But it took 21 years to get to that stage! We were told at three years old she was retarded! But I knew she was super clever at some things. She was putting sentences together at ten months and hasn't stopped talking since. (Parent)

My experience has been that parents who have had the best outcomes have been those with the confidence and ability to fight for what is their right. Challenging medical and educational professionals is something that many people do not feel comfortable with, but, sadly, is frequently necessary for parents of autistic females. For older women without parental support, the route to diagnosis is often a solitary one, sometimes met with resistance from professionals. At any age, it can be a dispiriting experience.

> Being an autistic parent to an autistic kid isn't hard, but the utter exhaustion when getting their needs met is, whether this be from social care, education or health. These providers need to listen and act. We know what our kids needs, and most of the time there isn't a big cost implication, just acceptance and understanding that all neurotypes are valuable and NDs [neurodivergents] are and have been imperative to world change.

In order to facilitate accurate diagnosis, it is important for parents and individuals themselves to refer to general autism behavioural characteristic lists and questionnaires focusing on the female behavioural profile (Attwood, 2013) and take copies of these with them to a diagnostic interview. The Internet is a great resource of behaviour checklists for the autism spectrum condition and there are many books available that outline what to expect. A note of caution, however: many online checklists of female autistic characteristics are much broader than the actual clinical diagnostic criteria. Anecdotally, these checklists have validity and report traits commonly seen in autistic females, but not all of the features listed will be considered in a diagnostic assessment. It is important to stick to the clinical criteria in order to ensure that these are met, otherwise there could be disappointment when the diagnosis is not given. Whether the current clinical diagnostic criteria are broad enough to encompass all autistic experience is another question, but for now, these are what autism is measured against and must be adhered to for a clinical autism outcome. Each item on the characteristics list or questionnaire should be fleshed out with specific examples of how the child/individual would meet each criterion. For an adult, evidence of childhood presentation is also recommended – school reports, photographs, conversations with family members and recollections from childhood help to form a lifelong picture. In essence, as a person seeking a diagnosis, you should provide as much evidence as possible to support your case to make the clinician's job as easy as possible. This is essential when seeking diagnosis for a female, whose outward presentation may not be sufficient for an uneducated, unwilling or inexperienced clinician.

The diagnostic criteria

> *I wouldn't want to see female specific diagnostic criteria, because a stereotypical male/female model is not helpful, and a more fluid approach is more useful. What we need to do is to listen with respect and without judgement. We need to believe what people tell us as clinicians and move away from stereotypical models of autism.*
>
> Dr Linda Buchan, Clinical Psychologist, Axia-ASD (2022)

Until recently, commonly used diagnostic criteria, such as the *Diagnostic and Statistical Manual of Mental Disorders* (DSM) and International Classification of Diseases (ICD), have not considered sex differences at all (Lord *et al.*, 1982; Gould and Ashton-Smith, 2011). The current DSM-5 criteria (American Psychiatric Association, 2013) show significant changes to the general criteria for autism spectrum disorders (ASDs) with the removal of independent diagnosis for Asperger syndrome and other changes to the required indicators. The criteria also mention sex differences for the first time, noting that diagnosed females tend to have accompanying intellectual disabilities, which implies that females of typical intellectual and language profiles – and consequently less visible differences – may not be identified as autistic.. Mandy (2013) adds his own comment on the potential implications of this:

> In this sense, the architects of the DSM-5 have laid down a

> challenge to researchers: Provide an account of the female phenotype, so that clinicians can learn to better identify, and help, females on the autism spectrum [without an accompanying intellectual disability].

The DSM-5 also includes the following new specifier, which may assist the female cause: 'Symptoms must be present in the early development period (but may not become fully manifest until social demands exceed limited capacities or may be masked by learned strategies in later life)' (American Psychiatric Association, 2013). The explicit recognition that autism may not be 'fully manifest' until life becomes unmanageable for an individual will, it is to be hoped, aid those seeking adult diagnosis who may, up until now, have been told: 'You can't have autism; you would have been diagnosed by now if you did'. Furthermore, the assertion that 'learned strategies' may be adopted, and the inference that they should be considered as part of the evidence of potentially autistic indicators, should not only aid more accurate diagnosis in both males and females, but also may have particular relevance to the documented masking abilities of females.

The DSM-5 criteria place a greater emphasis on restricted, stereotyped behaviours being observed, yet some research has found that autistic females do not exhibit these behaviours to the same degree as males, or at least not in the same way, which may exclude some females from receiving a diagnosis of ASD (Mandy *et al.*, 2012). Until new guidelines are developed that encompass female ASD, clinicians will have to fill in the gaps themselves, by developing a broader understanding of what to look for and who to listen to.

Many autism research professionals do not feel that the current non-gender specific criteria are necessarily in need of changing to better identify autism in females, but that the onus must be on clinicians to interpret them accurately with a good understanding of how autism may present in females. Dr Linda Buchan, director and clinical psychologist at Axia-ASD, agrees. She co-developed the Partnership Model of diagnosis, which sees the diagnostic process as a collaborative one between diagnostician and client, rather than a hierarchical one typically seen in clinical practice. The diagnostician-as-expert-based model is also redefined as seeing the client as the expert in themselves and their condition, which for females leads to a greater likelihood of their self-reported accounts of their lives being believed, rather than needing to be observed by a so-called 'expert' using prescriptive clinical tools which have not taken the female presentation into account. Dr Buchan feels that accurate diagnosis of females is less about a 'female profile' and more about viewing individuals in non-traditional ways.

Dr Buchan also notes the disparity between the profiles of those seeking assessment via UK NHS-funded referrals and those who have the financial means to self-fund their diagnosis. In her clinic, those from lower economic backgrounds and minority ethnic communities make up larger numbers of funded referrals, with the majority of self-funded referrals being from white, higher-economic backgrounds suggesting not only a potential gender bias in diagnosis, but also an economic and ethnic one too.

The diagnostic process

The diagnostic process itself takes a number of forms depending on the age and/or intellectual ability of the individual, and the clinical tools or process used by the diagnostic service or clinician. There is no definitive and objective test for autism and no standard way of carrying out an assessment. The outcome of the diagnostic assessment has a subjective element and is based on the quality and quantity of evidence gathered and the experience and opinion of the clinician or clinicians involved. Therefore, the knowledge and experience of the clinician is crucial in this process through both asking the right questions to elicit the necessary data and interpreting that data to provide an accurate outcome. For females this is even more important due to under-diagnosis, misdiagnosis, masking and differing presentation than traditionally seen in males, combined with the lottery of finding a clinician who knows what questions to ask and what to look for. Eileen Riley-Hall (2012) provides a detailed account in her book of the diagnostic process (in the US) that she went through with her two daughters. Following the diagnosis, professionals should have good knowledge of local referral points for services and links to information about understanding the diagnosis for both the individual and their family members. Diagnosis is only the beginning of the journey, not the end.

Most current diagnostic tools do not consider sex differences and only follow the diagnostic requirements as laid down by the DSM criteria. The likelihood of an accurate diagnosis for the individual is enhanced by the diagnostic processes and how clinicians are implementing them. If the tools are not accurate in identifying girls, then clinicians will have a hard job accurately assessing them. Frazier *et al.* (2014) suggests that sex-specific norms for some diagnostic processes might be helpful. The teaching of these methods should provide gender-differentiated examples to give new clinicians the breadth of presentation of the autistic profile. One review of health professionals engaged in the assessment of females found that the majority had received no training that addressed potential gender difference and were not adjusting their assessment practice in any way to taking gender into account; only 18.2 per cent of those asked were using female-specific measures (Freeman and Grigoriadis, 2023).

Another study (Cumin, Pelaez and Mottron, 2022) asked 20 diagnosticians how they conducted female autism assessments and collated their views into a series of statements. The participants noted that the Autism Diagnostic Observation Schedule version 2 (ADOS-2), a commonly used diagnostic tool, was ill equipped to detect autism in women without intellectual disability and resulted in false negatives. The ADOS-2 could also result in false positives where anxiety and mood disorders may skew results. Other features noted in autistic women that the participants considered diagnostically relevant were how they had often failed to achieve expected levels of professional or personal success and that peer relationships with neurotypical females were rare. The drive for seeking diagnosis was rarely for functional reasons but sought in order to understand themselves. Fluid and androgynous gender presentation was also observed. None of these features are mentioned in the current DSM diagnostic criteria but they go towards the development of a broad profile of the person and should lead to the clinician being alerted to possible autism.

In another study in which the ADOS-2 was tested, previously diagnosed autistic participants showed that it excluded autistic females at over 2.5 times the rate of excluding autistic males (D'Mello *et al.*, 2022) and yet, in the UK at least, it persists as the most commonly used clinical tool, which makes absolutely no sense at all. I sat through the ADOS-2 with a trainee psychologist several years ago as an opportunity for her to practise using it and for me to understand how it worked. In her opinion, she believed that I would have scored zero (a score of >30 is required for a diagnosis of autism). If by the end of this book you believe that I have zero autistic features, then perhaps the ADOS-2 is an accurate tool for adult females. Otherwise...I rest my case.

When training clinicians to use the Diagnostic Interview for Social and Communication Disorders (DISCO) assessment tool, Dr Judith Gould encourages them to examine the data gathered with a broader view:

> The criteria relate to the condition which are not gender specific. The point is how do clinicians interpret the criteria rather than changing the criteria? [...] The key is asking the right questions and sadly that only comes from experience and knowledge about the female presentation of the condition. Educating professionals as we do in our diagnostic training is one of the ways forward. (Gould, 2014)

Gould and Ashton-Smith (2011) also outline a number of key differences in autistic features between girls and boys and recommend a broader view of the diagnostic classification to be taken by clinicians. Items such as increased interest in reading fiction and immersing themselves in fantasy worlds (with set rules that can be followed) are mentioned as needing special consideration. It could be said that no clinician should diagnose (or rule out diagnosis of) autism in females without reference to sex-specific diagnostic materials such as these.

Self-reporting of autistic characteristics was also seen to be higher in women, despite fewer behaviours being observed when tested with clinical autism diagnostic tools (e.g. ADOS-2). This suggests that despite less obvious observable characteristics, women have the same (if not higher) perception of their autism, and its impact, as men. A first attempt has been made to develop a clinical self-report measure of autistic traits as described by autistic people (Ratto *et al.*, 2022). The Self-Assessment of Autistic Traits (SAAT) is intended for adults of all genders, and uses accessible language and a strength-based profile. The authors based their questionnaire on what autistic people said about autism and used autistic researchers to review and edit this. Autism research has largely focused on a deficit-based model of autistic experience, whereas in contrast, autistic people report positive aspects of their lives, which has thus far not been recognized. It is hoped by the authors that this preliminary version of the questionnaire will eventually be used as an adult screening tool in both diagnosis and research.

Tony Attwood and colleagues have developed screening tests for parents to support identification of autistic girls and studied the use of these as part of the diagnostic process for adult cis- and transwomen (Brown *et al.*, 2020). The questions focus on specifically female presentations of autism, such as gender toy preference, fantasy worlds and relationships with both people and animals. The test is used as part of a broader diagnostic assessment and at least begins to ask the right questions of parents in order to build a more accurate female profile. Assuming an obvious physical presentation of ASD in a female (or indeed in anyone) may be the first mistake made by an inexperienced clinician. A full picture of childhood behaviours, self-reports and cognitive assessments should form part of the process. There can be a tendency to ignore family and self-reporting, and for the clinician to prioritize what they can 'see', plus it has been suggested that parents may have higher expectations of the social and communication behaviour of girls than they do of boys and rate these accordingly, which may additionally skew any findings (McLennan, Lord and Schopler, 1993). Parents are not always experts in autism and will not know what relevant information to present during a diagnostic assessment. It is the clinician's role to prompt parents' recall in specific areas. Many of the questions asked in the Attwood screening test are not those commonly associated with male autism and are therefore not elements that a parent would necessarily think worthy of mentioning.

Diagnosis of adults and older people

Diagnosis may be more difficult for older people because they may not have living parents or family members to provide additional information relating to the childhood impact of autistic characteristics, which are required by some clinicians. I have worked with individuals who have been refused diagnosis on the grounds that they do not have a surviving parent. The *NICE Guidelines* (National Collaborating Centre for Mental Health, 2012) state that, 'where possible', a partner, family member or carer should be involved, but the lack of this information source is not grounds for refusing a diagnosis.

For those who do have living relatives, these relatives are likely to be very elderly themselves and may be unable to contribute. Other people may not wish to discuss the diagnosis with elderly parents for fear of upsetting them. Individuals may also have difficulty remembering significant details of childhood events and motivations and therefore struggle to demonstrate their early development. Current diagnostic tools are largely designed for the diagnosis of children and are therefore not appropriate for older people. Care must be taken when making a diagnosis of older women to take into account that they may have successfully developed compensating and masking strategies to hide their autism. Extensive experience of working with autistic adults is required to confidently and accurately diagnose older people and be able to 'see' the autism beneath the constructed social facade.

Some people question the point of diagnosis in later life, feeling that if a person has managed this far, then they can't be very affected or need a diagnosis.

> Getting a diagnosis is very difficult as there seems to be a school of thought that if you've survived with AS [Asperger syndrome] into your 40s, it can't be that bad (in fact there can be an enormous amount of suffering in silence).

Gender bias in female autism diagnosis

As previously mentioned, females are significantly less likely to receive a diagnosis than males (Giarelli *et al.*, 2010; Russell *et al.*, 2011), and by using current diagnostic methods, some females may 'look' less autistic but not actually 'be' or 'feel' any less autistic (Lai *et al.*, 2011). Girls and boys may be identified for diagnostic assessment at a similar age, but boys are more likely to receive an autism diagnosis whereas girls may receive a different diagnosis despite both sexes displaying markers/signs clinically associated with autism (Giarelli *et al.*, 2010). It may be that clinicians who are expecting autism to be more common in males are attributing certain behaviours to autism in boys and attributing the same behaviours to different conditions in girls. Equally, it may be that clinicians are expecting males and autistic females to behave in the same way, even though boys' and girls' behaviours are not considered to be identical in the typically developing population (McCarthy *et al.*, 2012; Ruigrok *et al.*, 2014). Head, McGillivray and Stokes (2014) studied social and emotional skills in males and autistic females and compared them to those in typically developing peers aged 12–16 years. They found that autistic females scored higher than autistic males, and at a similar level to typically developing males, but lower than typically developing females. They concluded that this could partly explain the potential under-diagnosis of females as social presentation is not currently gender-differentiated in the diagnostic criteria. They suggest that if an autistic female presents as more highly functioning than an autistic male, their abilities may appear superficially typical (and similar to that of a typical male) and therefore not be considered as notable if the clinician is using the male autistic social skills profile.

In children without an autism diagnosis, it is more common for girls to receive diagnoses of general developmental delay or seizure disorder – staring spells and seizure-like activity were five times more commonly diagnosed in girls than in boys (Giarelli *et al.*, 2010). Kopp and Gillberg (1992) report seeing many girls in their centre who 'do not clinically present the picture usually associated with autistic disorder' (p.90). These girls fulfil the criteria in childhood, but as they mature they present a considerably different profile to their male counterparts. Kopp and Gillberg (1992) suggest that some clinicians do not believe that these adult women could ever have fitted the full autistic profile earlier in life. A potential factor in these girls not presenting sufficiently to receive a positive diagnosis may be that the diagnostic criteria require responses to be made within a given time-frame. One of the noted issues for autistic girls is the length of time it takes them to respond socially – they may get there in the end but are noticeably slower than same-age peers (Nichols, Moravcik and Tetenbaum, 2009).

Missed and co-morbid diagnoses

Clinicians' attention can be diverted by the presentation of other co-morbid mental health conditions in teenage and adult life – conditions such as anorexia and anxiety disorders, which may be part of the autism profile but may not lead automatically to considering autism as the causal factor (Kopp and Gillberg, 1992; Simone, 2010). W. Lawson (2000) describes how it took 25 years to be diagnosed with Asperger syndrome after being wrongly diagnosed with schizophrenia. The majority of the women participants questioned for this book had experienced years of mental health difficulties (mainly anxiety) and interventions before receiving an autism diagnosis. Steph Jones, autistic therapist and author of *The Autistic Survival Guide to Therapy* (forthcoming) carried out an informal survey on Instagram of previous diagnoses given to autistic women, and responses included the usual suspects plus schizophrenia, attachment disorder and many more (Jones, pers. comm., 2023). A colleague of mine who works in a personality disorder service said that almost all of her female patients have emotionally unstable personality disorder (EUPD) diagnoses (another name for borderline personality disorder - BPD), and she believes that almost all of them would meet the criteria for autism at diagnosis, a process which she is committed to making accessible for them, should they wish it. Dr Linda Buchan, clinical psychologist at Axia-ASD diagnostic clinic, reports that EUPD/BPD is the most common misdiagnosis given to her female clients seeking autism assessment. She also notes that clinicians need to be able to disentangle trauma and autism; given that autistic people are more liable to experience trauma, it is necessary for clinicians to look for early childhood development prior to the trauma in order to make an accurate diagnosis. Clinicians agree that most adult autistic women have had trauma (Cumin *et al.*, 2022) and that attachment difficulties could resemble autism.

BPD may be wrongly given as a diagnosis as a result of autistic women finding similarly atypical peers who struggled to fit in, and associating in risky behaviours through them as a result of mimicking them (Cumin *et al.*, 2022). In order to differentiate between the two conditions, those with BPD typically have no differences in social communication when in a period of stability, whereas this would be a consistent feature of autism. Women with BPD can also typically name, express and explain their emotions easily, while autistic women find this hard, sometimes due to accompanying alexithymia. Women with BPD also tend to note fear of abandonment as a problem; autistic women are more likely to need to be alone.

> [It took] five years or so to finally pinpoint the condition after I scored highly positive in a preliminary written questionnaire regarding AS [Asperger syndrome]. The difficulty came in my other issues obfuscating the root cause of my behaviourisms. I've been called anywhere from bipolar to schizophrenic and have had medication provided thusly to combat those symptoms.

> I have been misdiagnosed most of my life, including hearing doctors tell my mother that I had emotional problems, that I was trying to get attention, that I had nervous problems or that I was neurotic. Later I was diagnosed with learning disabilities in high school. In college, a doctor who initially thought I was psychotic eventually diagnosed me as having severe neurosis with schizoid tendencies.

> Looking back at my diagnosis, the psychiatrist also diagnosed me as having anankastic personality disorder or obsessive-compulsive personality disorder; [it] seems very interesting to me that she picked up what were a lot autistic traits but gave me that diagnosis instead of questioning autism itself.

> I was misdiagnosed with borderline personality disorder, which seemed to fit at the time as my life seemed to be one mental health crisis after another.

Nichols *et al.* (2009) suggest that routes to eventual autism diagnosis for a female can include the following steps, and that a fuller knowledge and understanding of these can aid the clinician in considering autism when assessing the person and can potentially facilitate more accurate diagnosis:

- previous diagnosis of another disorder or several disorders, including attention deficit hyperactivity disorder (ADHD), anxiety, depression, obsessive-compulsive disorder and eating disorders (Nichols *et al.* (2009) suggest that the older the girl, the more diagnoses she is likely to have collected)
- a diagnosis of social anxiety or general difficulty in social situations
- adult women with a previous diagnosis of schizophrenia or psychotic disorder
- another family member with an ASD diagnosis

- presentation or apparent deterioration of capacity to cope as adolescence approaches, where social relationships become more nuanced and complex (in adolescence, girls may not demonstrate typically 'female' social interests, such as fashion and relationships).

An inexperienced clinician's 'tick-box' approach to the autism diagnostic criteria may be very harmful to individuals with a different behavioural profile. An extensive knowledge of autism and face-to-face experience of a significant number of autistic women are necessary. Reading autobiographies, blogs, watching YouTube videos made by autistic women and spending a day or two at a special school or women's support group will all help to build the real-life knowledge essential to be a competent clinician.

Benefits in diagnosis

> I was told repeatedly by many professionals that I did not *need* a diagnosis, but I always felt not fully believed and having to justify myself without one.

> I would get angry sometimes about the environment: 'Why is everyone being so loud? Why are the lights so bright?... they should know, this is horrible'. [Now, it's] like 'oh, no one else can hear that!' (Neville, 2019, p.24)

For either the parents of a child or the adult themselves, a positive diagnosis of autism is the start of a new journey of understanding, acceptance and adjusted expectations. The diagnosis is the key to progress for the individual and their family, and the benefits extend beyond the 'medical' explanation. The importance of a timely diagnosis cannot be over-emphasized, especially for those who may require – now or in their future lives – formalized support and accommodations. Neville (2019) found that the diagnosis of autism was a 'pivotal moment in empowering' (p.25) the adult women in her study to more effectively manage their own well-being.

Following diagnosis, psychologically, the family or individual now know what they are facing, so they can move on and deal with it (Eaton, 2012). Emotions can be mixed with sadness, guilt and anger, intermittently entwined with relief, acceptance and hope. The reported additional difficulty that females may have had in obtaining the appropriate diagnosis can make these feelings especially intense. The need to be heard and taken seriously is something shared by many parents of children and adult women on the autism spectrum. The successful diagnosis is evidence that this has happened. The 'vindication' that adult women describe attests to the intensity of this emotion and the importance of diagnosis.

> I hope that armed with this self-knowledge and awareness, the second half of my life will be more productive, fruitful and honest than the first, and that I will no longer feel worthless, stupid and useless and a failure in life. In addition, I wanted to be able to guide my children through their lives in a way that was not available to me. [...] I have begun a journey of self-acceptance and discovery. I am learning who I am and peeling away years of armour and masks to reveal the true essence of the person underneath. I try to be more assertive when negotiating for the small things that make navigating this life easier and am less apologetic for my quirkiness and differences that people find so unusual.

Families see one of the major benefits of a child receiving a diagnosis is that it formalizes and kick-starts a support process. Families also mention reflecting on their parenting methods and understanding the need to modify these in light of the confirmation of autism. For the families who participated in my research, the diagnosis brought a new and positive sense of direction to their attitude towards their children's care.

> We have stopped trying to use conventional behaviour techniques and adapted them to work; [now we understand] why they weren't working in the first place. Mostly, it meant, as parents, we could stop beating ourselves with the 'bad parenting' stick that many people (professional and otherwise) are eager to wield when behaviour is atypical (at best) and dangerous (at worst). (Parent)

> The difference was probably greatest for the family in a psychological sense. We had all been kidding ourselves that she was probably just a bit neurotic and intelligent. When she scored so highly on the ADOS-2 [autism diagnostic tool] it came as a bit of a shock to realize that she was actually quite severely affected in many ways. It has helped us understand and empathize with her better. And it has shut up other members of the family who were convinced she was just 'difficult'! (Parent)

Current thinking suggests that early diagnosis, and therefore appropriate support and intervention, are in the best interests of autistic individuals. The later-diagnosed adult women questioned had varying responses, with the majority feeling that an earlier diagnosis could have given them access to opportunities that had been denied to them due to an inability to access support; they also felt it could have saved them from a lot of emotional pain and the feeling that there was something very wrong with them. Interestingly, several adult-diagnosed women said they would have liked to have been diagnosed earlier than they were, but not necessarily in childhood. They felt that a childhood diagnosis may have resulted in limitations being placed on them by themselves and also by others in their lives – parents and teachers – who may have tried to protect them.

> I would definitely have liked to have been diagnosed earlier. I spent the first 13 years of my life thinking I was nothing but a freak (that mindset still sticks with me today), simply because that's how the world viewed me.

> I feel I have sacrificed the gifts from my Aspieness in order to fit in. Maybe if I had been diagnosed earlier I would not have spent a whole life trying to fit in, and would have been able to forgive my own social deficits, thus saving the energy and intellect required to pretend to be normal, which I could have dedicated to things that I really wanted to do, such as research into science and/or languages.

> It would've changed my entire life, in short. It wouldn't have allowed my chronic depression, which coincided with my not knowing what was 'wrong' with me during that crucial time of my life, to overwhelm me or leave me awash with the cycle of perpetual procrastination that it did. It condemned me to an abyss of endless inaction. I still resent those more professional people around me for not spotting the signs sooner.

Some adult-diagnosed women feel great regret and sadness at the opportunities missed and lost through not knowing. For some this can lead to feelings of bitterness and blame towards those who did not support them, especially with parents who may have been unknowingly autistic themselves. In some cases, this may be justified, but often it is simply a matter of being born too early for the awareness to have been even possible. Managing these feelings through therapy or self-reflection can be useful in being able to move on from this sense of being wronged, which can become all-consuming and damaging to those relationships concerned and mental health in general.

Women who commented that they would not have wanted an earlier diagnosis felt that they were stronger and more capable because of what they had been through. Some of them felt that children diagnosed nowadays are sometimes overprotected and, as a result, are less independent than they were.

> Positives would have been maybe getting some help, support and understanding. Negatives would have been having my

> aspirations downgraded – you can't manage that, it would be too stressful, etc., and seeing yourself as 'less' and defective.

> [Maybe] but any early intervention/help may ultimately have hindered my development into the adult I've become – I believe I'm stronger through having struggled at times and am far more prepared for the nature of adult life than some people who have had support for years.

> I probably wouldn't have been nearly so independent and self-reliant as I am today [...] When I see so many young people with Asperger's who seem to be so protected (by their mums especially), I don't think it's good for them. I think the parents don't realize how much their son or daughter could do if they were encouraged more instead of being made to feel they are disabled.

Fortunately, girls and young women today have awareness on their side, and for them early diagnosis is a positive outcome that may protect them from some of the ancillary mental health issues experienced by older women and equip them with the understanding that they are capable of anything they choose. The support is there for them. Many of the young women I meet in colleges around the country, where I work, are comfortable with their autism; it's no big deal – they've had it forever. They don't want to talk about it; they just get on with it. It's a totally different experience to the late-diagnosed adult women coming to the realization for the first time: we want to talk about it, dissect it, analyse it.

Dr Catriona Stewart OBE (2022) sees that young women who have known that they are autistic since childhood have greater self-awareness and are better able to identify their own needs and look after themselves. Masking for these young women still happens but is less damaging. She also notes that younger autistic girls can be at severe risk of harm to their mental health due to being overwhelmed at school without the support a diagnosis can bring. She says:

> These girls have the ability to be assertive and are the most amazing human beings. All the odds are stacked up against them and yet they are incredibly resilient. It is important that we don't give these young women a negative narrative of life as an autistic person which can lead to them being over-protected. They mustn't restrict themselves to anything they have been told about autism.

For many adult women, self-diagnosis is an increasingly accepted concept. For various reasons, which may include financial considerations and access to diagnostic providers that women trust, formal diagnosis is unobtainable. For those that seek some form of external autism assessment, their stated reasons for doing so include words such as 'permission', 'validation' and 'confirmation'. They often express a great certainty in their belief that they are autistic, and have spent many hours researching the subject before drawing this conclusion, but feel that they need an 'official' verification before being able to disclose to others and to put in place approaches that will allow them to live more autistically. Self-doubt and a fear of the doubt of others seem to play a large part in needing a diagnosis in order to have the confidence to make it public, or even fully internalize it themselves. Others express a need for a yes/no answer, having had the unresolved notion of 'Am I/Aren't I autistic?' for a long time. There is no irony in the binary nature of the autistic mind seeking definitive certainty.

> My head had been spinning all my life with trying to make sense of why these things happened to me, why I was so odd, why I couldn't live like other people. The diagnosis stopped my head from spinning. I was able to breathe a sigh of relief and relax.

Benefits for formally diagnosed individuals include being able to access practical support and being taken more seriously by service providers.

> It allowed for suitable housing to be gained, benefits to be

> granted, and a level of explanation I could offer the banks, etc. for the out-of-control finances and other severe problems our daughter had at the time. The full weight of the situation began to shift [from being] purely [on] my shoulders, as the mum, to a shared level with others. We were granted 10½-hours-a-week support – life changing for me! (Parent)

What some people find frustrating, however, is that frequently specialist knowledge stops at the point of diagnosis (Eaton, 2012), leaving individuals and families without significant follow-up support or expertise from then onwards. Sadly, resources for these services appear to be increasingly scarce, and the only option for many people is to fund this support themselves, which means that it is only available to those with sufficient financial means to do so. For many autistic people – given health and employment impacts – this is out of the question. Although, conversely, for those who can afford to pay for support, the number of (mostly female) autistic therapists is greater than ever before, allowing the possibility at least of support from someone who truly understands the female autistic perspective.

Post-diagnostic disclosure

> It's always a tricky balance because revealing you're autistic relies on the person you're disclosing to knowing what that means.

Once the diagnosis of autism has been confirmed, the process of deciding who to tell and how to tell other people begins. Some find that becoming an advocate for autism is a role that they feel comfortable with, celebrating their own or their child's unique self and sharing their knowledge to increase understanding in others. Liane Holliday Willey is an advocate of full disclosure and writes a chapter on it in her book *Pretending to be Normal* (2014), which beautifully portrays the mind of an autistic woman – a must-read for all clinicians and practitioners. For parents, this may mean that they can gain some tolerance for their child's behaviour when things get difficult.

> When we are out and about, my husband and I will explain to people she [autistic daughter] makes a bee-line for before they have a chance to make judgements (e.g. in restaurants, she will go over and talk to people at their tables and doesn't read the social cues for when they've had enough), and usually this makes people really tolerant and, as she is very endearing, they usually have a lovely interaction. (Parent)

Surprise and disbelief at the diagnosis cropped up frequently for the participants in this book as reactions to their disclosure. This was either because they were girls, or because they 'looked too normal'.

> One person told me, 'I thought that autistic people were retarded and couldn't speak'.

> I get told I'm brave occasionally – which I hate, because to be brave there must have been a reason to be afraid, and that suggests I've missed a fear I should have had. I'm not brave for being autistic or disclosing I'm autistic; I'm just a person trying to get through life as best she can.

> The other friend began treating me like a person with a very low IQ, doing up my coat if it was cold out, answering for me if I was asked a question, making decisions on my behalf, repeatedly asking me if I was okay, etc. It made me feel uncomfortable and slightly ridiculous.

> I told people I suspected it was ASD and I got lots of raised eyebrows and 'she's not because she gives eye contact / her language is great/she doesn't flap or rock, etc.' but once we had the diagnosis, people were more willing to listen to how girls present very differently. (Parent)

> I had mentioned to two counsellors and a psychotherapist previously that I thought I may be autistic and been laughed at (literally) because I was a trained counsellor and had a 'normal' life.

> I have had some irritating responses, such as 'you're not very autistic', 'you can't use that as an excuse for everything' and 'we're all a little bit autistic'.

The perception that if the presentation isn't immediately visible then the autism isn't something requiring accommodation is a common, but often incorrect, one. This can make it feel difficult and disappointing for some women to reveal this new and precious discovery, which for many has changed their lives, only for it to be dismissed without care. What is important, in my opinion, is that you do not feel that you have to justify 'how' autistic you are in the face of their doubt. If someone says that you 'can't be autistic' or 'we are all a bit like that', I suggest simply smiling, nodding and saying nothing. Give it a try and watch what happens!

When advising newly diagnosed individuals on how they may share this new knowledge with those close to them, I first advise them to wait – for days, weeks or months even. There can be quite an emotional rollercoaster of joy, sadness, anger, grief and more, and I believe that it is important to allow some of that to settle before exposing oneself to the well-meaning ignorance of others. Once you have revealed being autistic, you cannot then take that back and ever be seen as you were previously. You may later decide that you prefer to be more selective about who you tell, but at that point, it will be too late.

It is also, in my opinion, necessary to try to see things from the perspective of those on the receiving end of your news. These may be people who have known you for many years, and due to their own lack of understanding (and remember that you probably shared this lack only a short time ago before autism came into your world and you had devoured every blog, podcast, book and video on the subject) may be entirely unable to believe that you could fit their perceived view of what autism is. Their view is likely to consider not only that being autistic is impossible in your case, but also that even if it were possible, then it is a tragedy or at the very least not a good thing. If it is your parents or close family members that you are disclosing to, they may also have some sense of sadness or guilt that you may have suffered or feel that they are being blamed. This discomfort can sometimes make people feel defensive or attacked and want to make that discomfort go away by denying the existence of its cause. These factors combined make it highly likely that at least some people that you tell will immediately refute your disclosure and try to reassure you that this cannot possibly be the case. The idea that discovering you are autistic is the best thing that has ever happened to you would not be on their radar (unless they are autistic too).

If it is important to you that people understand how you feel about the diagnosis and respond accordingly, I would advise telling them how you feel about the information that you are just about to share with them – before you share it with them. Something like:

> I have something important to tell you and I want you to hear what I have to say and listen to my feelings about it. This event has been very positive for me, and I am entirely sure that it is correct. I want you to accept what I have to say in those terms, rather than express doubt or sympathy.

I would also advise on selecting a short video clip or passage of text which encapsulates your autistic experience and one which your intended listener could identity you with. This can help to externally validate your disclosure in their eyes. In the case of parents, some reassurance that they are not to blame, and an explanation of how it may not have been possible for them to have known (due to historical factors), may also be helpful and kind. Appreciating that you are not the only person who may have an emotional reaction to this diagnosis, and that it is very unlikely that they will be able to empathize with your positive feelings about it (again, unless they are autistic), can lead to a more positive reception.

Adult discovery and diagnosis

> I realize that the first year post-diagnosis I was obsessed by the topic but now it's just no longer a special interest and on some days I'd be happy if I never heard the word again. I suppose it's like eating too much chocolate cake!

> There are thousands of us – women who discovered our autism well into adulthood – well past many of the memories it explains. We're too late in life to prevent a multitude of misunderstandings, yet too early in history to say, 'I'm autistic!' and trust that everyone will know what we mean. We need to unpuzzle the past to heal our hearts, and the present to see who we are. (Kotowicz, 2022, p.1)

Many of the women I questioned had received their diagnosis of autism after their teenage years, some not until much later. Some of these women had spent the vast majority of their lives not knowing that they were autistic and having no self-awareness and no support. Due to the point in history that they were born, they grew up in a time when only children (and only male ones at that) could be autistic; they had to find their own way, often experiencing major crises and challenges along the way. Their lives were full of observations about their perceived differences, usually with no explanation for these apparent anomalies and contradictions involving their uneven skill profiles, challenges and unique quirks.

> We can read books and understand anything written better than most but can't follow social conversation. We can dismantle computers and install hardware but can't find our way around a supermarket. We can monologue for hours on our special interests but can't spend an hour in conversation without getting a migraine or having a meltdown. We can paint pictures and design things of astonishing beauty but can't be bothered to fix our own hair. (Simone, 2010, p.211)

> I have always been thrown by people asking, 'How are you?' because I thought they wanted a real answer, and I would talk for far too long. Even now, I have to school myself to just say, 'Fine. How are you?' But I often forget and find myself talking about myself...for a good five minutes before I remember that I should have just said 'Fine'.

> When someone asks: 'What's happening?' I don't really know what I'm supposed to say. Do I tell them how my entire day was? Or what is happening in the world? Or what is happening at my house? Or with my daughter? Or is it just code for 'hello'? Each time I eventually decide it must be code for 'hello', but then I forget about that decision when I hear it a few weeks later and go through the entire thought process again. I'm hoping that next time I will remember that it is just code for 'hello' – because I looked it up as part of writing this.

The sense of difference that many women feel, I believe, stems from this uneven profile. It makes it very hard to work out where you belong when you are brilliant at things that others find hard, but useless at things that others find easy. This is why the diagnosis, at any age, can come as such a relief. It explains everything. It makes sense of everything. And autistic women need to make sense of everything.

> Where do I belong? Wherever you go, whatever you do, whoever you are, you never fit in. This is about wanting to find your home. (Stewart, 2022)

> Every once in a while, I would spot a stranger, or sometimes a minor character in a movie or play, and imagine that she might be one of the humans who felt like me. I imagined us having similar motivations, reactions, memories and perspectives. I had a word for such people – a 'Me'. I would see them and think to myself, 'I wonder if she's a Me?' (Kotowicz, 2022, p.6)

One of the most common things I am asked when discussing diagnosis for autistic adults is: 'What's the point?' The presumption is that if you have made it to 40 or 50 years of age without a diagnosis and survived, why bother getting one now? As one woman puts it:

> It put many of the difficulties I had with school and friendships into perspective, as well as allowing me to work out why I find some situations very stressful/tiring (social occasions, meeting new people, loud environments, etc). [...] In short, it was a massive relief – I know who I am, how I can expect myself to be, that there's nothing 'wrong' with me, and that the friendship difficulties I had weren't my fault.

Women receiving late diagnosis often share the same sense of relief and self-acceptance as men, but perhaps to an even greater degree, due to the way in which they have needed to manage their autism – often through bending to fit to what's expected of them in terms of gender expectations through camouflaging (which autistic men are seen as less prone to and/or able to do). Feeling justified or vindicated by diagnosis is the strong response of many of the women I have spoken to: a sense of having the right to be yourself established – for the first time – in a world that doesn't always welcome or appreciate that self. These are women who are exhausted and angry at having tried so hard to make everything make sense, while presuming that they were to blame for not getting it in the first place: women who feel they have had to put on a persona of social acceptability in order to be tolerated. I often see individuals go through a phase of what I call 'militant' autism following diagnosis, where the person decides to behave exactly as they please, almost as a knee-jerk response to rejecting their former existence. For most people, this is part of the post-diagnostic process of coming to terms with what this new information means, and a more moderate position on how to exist more happily is usually found over time. When asked what difference having an adult diagnosis meant for them, common themes are self-acceptance and being kinder to oneself.

> Getting diagnosed has been one of the most meaningful experiences of my life because it has made sense of everything.

> I went through a grieving process I think, for the allistic [not on the autism spectrum] person I had pretended to be for 40 years; my partner and family didn't respond well to my diagnosis, and I was depressed about it for a while.

> Being told I was autistic felt like being given a key to the rest of my life.

> It was as important a moment in my life as the birth of my children.

> I literally feel like I've been reborn. I'm so much kinder to myself now I'm out of the neurotypical hamster wheel of trying to keep up. It has completely changed my life.

> The clouds parted and the angels sang. Even before I got the official diagnosis, something just *clicked* inside me. Suddenly all the places I thought I was broken, all the ways I'd 'failed' to be a normal human, just didn't matter. I wasn't broken or failed (or moody or sensitive or aggressive or prickly or annoying or weird): I was autistic. (Schembari, 2023)

> I felt immensely proud of myself for coping as well as I have. It changed my perspective from 'I haven't coped well in life' to 'I have coped extremely well in life'.

When working with newly diagnosed women, I describe the diagnosis as a new framework for making sense of what works and what doesn't, and how the value of the diagnosis is in putting this new understanding into practice in order to create or tweak a life which maximizes joy and minimizes stress and overwhelm. The commitment to making practical use of this new survival manual has led to some women making enormous changes to their lives (who said we didn't like change?!). These are pragmatic individuals who, when given the right instructions, will go to great lengths to 'fix' the problem of trying to be 'normal' by making their own path.

> Since diagnosis I have changed careers, moved to live in the middle of nowhere, I work from home, I work compressed hours, I live a life that suits me perfectly, and when I get the balance right I have more than enough energy to do the things I enjoy doing, alongside being a mum and working full time.

> My life is unrecognisable to how it was before. I found out how to be happy and embraced it.

> I have plans that are based on who I am, rather than who I think I ought to be. I spent my first half-century trying to fit in and now I have stopped. If anyone questions my oddness, I tell them it's because I'm odd. (National Autistic Society, 2013a)

> [...]A massive difference, mainly in terms of understanding myself and not being so hard on myself. It explained so much of my life, my needs, my choices, and it made me feel justified and validated in being how I am. It makes it easier to meet people and take on new experiences because I know why I find things difficult; I know what might help, and if it doesn't work, I am more accepting.

> The first thing to change was my relationship with my daughter. Before my diagnosis I was an angry mom with a rage problem. I was constantly yelling at my kid because I was constantly overstimulated. I thought I *had* to push through because I saw other moms able to do these things. But once I learned I was autistic, I was able to make small accommodations for myself I had never even considered before... I often screamed at my daughter... because she would talk while the radio was playing. I didn't realize trying to filter all that noise was flooding my system... After

> my diagnosis I realized what had been happening. Every time my daughter wanted to talk to me, I would turn off the radio. So simple, but so life-changing. Now we have a 'rule' where you can't talk to mommy if you have the radio on or a movie playing. That simple change has meant I so rarely yell at my daughter any more. I can't even remember the last time I did that, that's how long it's been.

Mostly the women felt happy to be autistic and had no desire to be different, despite the challenges they had faced. It must be noted that the type of person who willingly contributes to autism research such as this is more likely to be someone who is aware and knowledgeable about their condition, and perhaps is more likely to feel positive about it than someone less educated about it. In some of the women, pride in their identity and, dare I say it, contempt for NT values, are evident.

> [...]No, because then I wouldn't be me. You don't take off the autistic part and discover a 'normal' person underneath. I am autistic the way you have blue eyes or curly hair. It goes all the way through, like letters in seaside rock. It governs the way I think, listen to my body, the way my body talks back to me, how I see the world, everything.

> I am glad that I have autism; I find the NTs confusing, like sheep following each other around. They never seem to say what they mean. I try to avoid them.

> I am proud to be autistic [...] [Looking objectively at NTs] Yes, some are good, but many routinely tell lies, exclude those who are different, subscribe to superficial trends, talk nonsense and are obsessed with conformity. Why would I want to be NT? Ugh.

> Autism makes me very unique, and in principle I don't mind being different. I know I am very capable and very intelligent in

> a unique way. I just wish I had the social skills to be able to do something good with that set of skills.

And so, we can see the life-changing nature of this discovery for both parents and adult females themselves. It opens the door to understand how to create the best possible life for the individual rather than operating through trial and error in the dark. It gives the instruction manual, the guidebook and the operating procedures, and that for many is a huge relief in itself. Next we take a look at exactly what it is that defines a person as autistic.

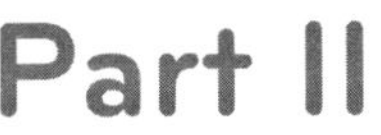

Part II

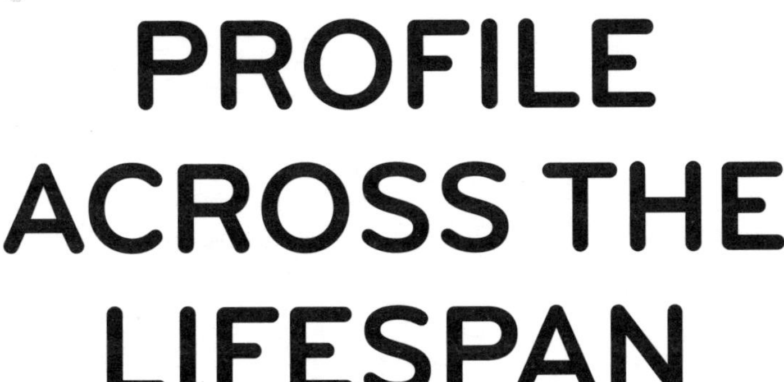

PROFILE ACROSS THE LIFESPAN

Chapter 3

INFANCY AND CHILDHOOD

> *By the time I was three years old, my parents knew I was not an average child.*
>
> Liane Holliday Willey (2014, p.18)

Parents whose daughters receive a diagnosis of autism later in life often say that they 'just knew' something was different about their child when she was a baby, or certainly often from a very early age – well before any current formal indicators of diagnosis could possibly be used. If the child has a language or developmental delay, it is more likely that the diagnosis of autism will occur sooner rather than later. The child will alert professional attention due to their lack of reaching early childhood milestones, rather than necessarily any specific autistic behaviour. The autism diagnosis may come at the same time – sometimes as young as two years of age – but often the conclusive diagnosis of an autism spectrum disorder (ASD) is reserved until an older age to ensure that the assessment is correct and consistent over time and natural development. For families with no knowledge or understanding of autism, this can at first be a huge shock and feel like the end of the world.

> We had our suspicions very early on, when my daughter was a young baby, that something was amiss. She didn't smile until much later than her peers, could not instinctively play with peers,

> [was] very socially awkward, [and had] poor gross and fine motor control, etc. But she was very bright verbally and taught herself to read when she was about three. We knew nothing about autism then and it seemed like a horrific condition. A teacher suggested it when my daughter was about six and we threw up our hands in horror. (Parent)

For children who do not have any learning disability or language delay, a diagnosis of autism would not necessarily be an obvious conclusion under three or four years of age, and therefore it is to be expected that diagnosis for these children would come later. This seems to be particularly the case with girls. One study found the average age of diagnosis in girls to be eight years of age (Eaton, 2012). Giarelli *et al.* (2010) found that boys were more likely to be given an ASD diagnosis earlier than girls, despite both sexes being identified as having similar language and developmental delays at approximately the same age. The girls were initially given a diagnosis of another condition, meaning that the commencement of appropriate support was delayed. A large-scale study of more than 20,000 females found that they were typically diagnosed 14 months later than males (Kavanaugh *et al.*, 2023). Reasons for this included limited repetitive behaviours, 'mild or atypical presentation' and intact IQ and language, with symptoms emerging later in development.

In my participant sample, the earliest diagnosis was at four years of age for a girl with an intellectual disability, while others without such an intellectual disability were slightly older. It is encouraging to learn that some clinicians are identifying ASD so early in these girls and clearly have a good understanding of how to interpret the diagnostic criteria for the female population. For the parents of these children there is often not anything 'wrong' with their child that they can define or that requires medical assistance, but more a nagging sense of something being different that they can't quite put their finger on. It might be that play is different, or that the child appears unusually absorbed and in a world of their own (Riley-Hall, 2012). This is particularly the case for parents of autistic girls as their behaviour may just be attributed by others as 'shy' (Kreiser and White, 2014) in a way that often isn't the case with boys. In my experience, these parents are frequently correct in their intuition, but can often be assumed to be over-anxious or imagining things. Obviously, it is not currently appropriate to make a very early autism diagnosis in all cases, but it may be necessary to note the observations of parents voicing concerns of this nature as at some point in the future this could potentially provide valuable supporting evidence for an autism diagnosis. One girl even had the insight to diagnose herself!

> By age eight she was questioning if she was on the autistic spectrum herself. We had already been asking [professionals] and had been fobbed off with the fact she was a girl! Her brother started going through the diagnostic process when she was eight and he was six. By the time she was nine he had been diagnosed with AS [Asperger syndrome] and she was convinced she was AS too [...] (took another 12 years!). (Parent)

> At age 13 years...we noticed she wasn't as sociable as her friends. By 15 years, she started having the odd day off school. We knew something was wrong but didn't expect the cause to be autism. It was only during an orthodontic appointment when our daughter was very uncomfortable with the treatment and the orthodontist remarked 'Is she autistic?' that the penny started to drop, and we started to explore autism. (Parent)

Childhood indicators

> From birth she was quite plainly different, but I hadn't any experience to base anything on until I started to study it myself. (Milner *et al.*, 2019)

> My kindergarten suggested I get assessed, and I was deemed retarded as I wouldn't participate in the stupid assessment

> which was done in baby talk and baby games. They ignored the fact I could already play chess and read books considered too advanced for me. (Baldwin and Costley, 2016, p.487)

When considering typical expected behaviours of an autistic child, parents of girls and autistic women give us an insight into their world in these early years. Some of the behaviours are not gender-specific and will also be seen in boys, particularly at this early stage, but expectations of how girls 'should' be may impact on how these pre-diagnosis behaviours are interpreted. It is important that autism remains on the radar when considering the causes of certain behaviours in these girls. We should remember that mental health or more general global-delay-type diagnoses are known to be more readily given to females when autism may have been more appropriate. Parents' observations about their children's behaviours are frequently made with hindsight; they may have caused concern at the time, but parents often fear being told they are paranoid or over-anxious, and keep these niggles to themselves. On reflection, the parents questioned had all noticed early atypical behaviour in their infants and toddlers, which later contributed to the picture they now know to be autism. One large-scale review of literature on the subject of early childhood signs of autism in females from ages 0 to 6 years found that there were more sex/gender similarities than differences in these early years (Chellew, Barbaro and Freeman, 2022). Differences found related to females making more repetitive movements, having a more advanced vocabulary, having less interest in parts of mechanical objects, and being more likely to engage in complex imitation than their male peers.

Typical very early indicators and parental anecdotal reports relate to characteristics and behaviours that include the following:

- the parent feels a sense of detachment from the baby or young child – often this cannot be further articulated by the parent; it is just a feeling of the baby or child 'being in their own world'
- atypical eye contact (either unusually limited or staring)

- a lack of attention paid specifically to people and faces – interest in people is not prioritized over objects
- limited interest and/or response to people stimuli (smiling, voices, peek-a-boo games)
- limited reciprocal social facial expressions and social cues (smiling, pointing)
- limited seeking-out of people and responses from people
- very placid, silent and peaceful babies – 'It was spooky... almost as though she was a ghost just lying there silently without moving' (parent)

OR

- very anxious, distressed and clingy babies – 'Intense emotions, especially distress, and an inability to be comforted by affection' (Attwood, 2012)
- sensory preferences and intolerances:
  - small temperature tolerance range, which can result in febrile convulsions
  - clothing (texture and touch)
  - physical touch (distressed by being cuddled)
  - specific and strong food preferences and dislikes
  - food and other intolerances and allergies.

Professor Tony Attwood has developed a Girls' Questionnaire for Autism Spectrum Conditions (GQ-ASC) (Attwood, 2013) for use by clinicians with parents of girls seeking diagnosis, to highlight female-specific characteristics and ensure that a full and accurate profile is provided. This tool is not a diagnostic test for autism in its own right but rather a supplementary information source asking the right questions to get the right information. The questions include items such as toy preference, imaginary friends/animals, adopting personas in different situations and responses to social errors. All of the items on Attwood's screening questionnaire were evidenced in the girls and women questioned for this book and are aspects of autism not usually considered indicative in traditional diagnostic measures.

As we have learned, autistic girls can often do a great job of masking their differences through rote learning and mimicking (typically) intuitive communication cues in order to pull off an effective social performance. However, at a young age, it is unlikely that this learning will be fully embedded and so any difference in social engagement should be evident. It may not be until the child joins a nursery or playgroup that the parent realizes that their 'quirky' child is really quite different from her peers. Preferences and behaviour, which in isolation at home are easily managed, may not be so easily accepted in a room full of 20 toddlers. It also may not be until the start of group interaction in formal play settings that the child begins to struggle with the more frequent and numerous social interactions and requirements. Therefore, a child who displayed few difficulties at home may suddenly appear much more affected by potential autism due to the change in her environment and the new expectations placed on her – and this may be particularly the case for girls who may be encouraged towards pretend, group and imaginative play in these settings.

Participants in the research for this book were asked for examples of early atypical behaviours that reflect behaviours associated with the autism diagnostic criteria, along with those identified as being potentially more indicative of female autism. The list of topics featured here is not exhaustive and is not a comprehensive list of diagnostic characteristics. They are topics that came up most frequently in my research and also in that of others as being particularly pertinent for these girls and women.

Non-verbal communication

Differences with the expression and reading of non-verbal signals, such as eye contact, facial expressions, tone of voice and body language, are presumed to be the more obvious and visible characteristics of autism. Autistic girls show 'clear limitations' in socio-emotional reciprocal behaviour. Their reciprocity skills are higher than for autistic boys but show 'subtle differences' when compared to typically developing girls (Backer van Ommeren *et al.*, 2016). Autistic girls made more social gestures than autistic boys, but also more errors in identifying emotions from faces. This use of gestures may be indicative of camouflaging and lead to a risk of under-diagnosis (Rynkiewicz *et al.*, 2016). It must be remembered that these are reciprocal skills in typically developing children, which result in the ability not only to 'read' other people, but also to present the appropriate non-verbal signals to enable other people to 'read' them. The autistic child may fail not only to pick up on cues from others and respond to those, but also to make the necessary facial expressions to transmit their own messages outwards to be received by others. Thus, a child who makes few facial expressions, or ones that appear slightly out of context in the situation, is certainly a candidate for consideration of autism in the same way as a child who does not actively respond to cues.

> On holiday aged eight, a kindly hotel owner observed that I never smiled and asked why I always looked so worried. I panicked as I didn't know what to answer, so I came out with the first thing that seemed reasonable to be worried about, which was 'the ozone layer'. I must have heard about this on the news.

Eye contact was mentioned by parents of autistic girls as being noticeably different in infancy in their daughters. This is something that is typically observed in babies within the first few weeks of life (assuming there are no physical visual problems). Eye contact differences in autistic individuals can range from little or no eye contact through to staring. The difference for an autistic person is in the intuitive understanding of eye contact as a means of reciprocal communication (and therefore not discerning any function in looking at someone's eyes), a difficulty in attending to more than one sensory input at once, or simply an intense discomfort at the intensity of looking into another person's eyes. As an adult, an autistic person may observe that eye contact is a social norm and teach themselves to replicate this (with varying levels of success), while a small child is behaving in their natural state, rather than one with learned modifications.

> While breastfeeding she would pull away if I gazed at her. While in her door-bouncer she would turn around to face the opposite direction if I tried to engage with her. (Parent)

> I have quite a number of memories that date back to two years of age and onward. Most of my memories of people during my toddler years are of parts of their bodies and not their faces or eyes (e.g. feet, hands, hair).

It is important to note that in autism a lack of eye contact does not equate to someone not understanding or listening. This may give rise to a child being described as a 'daydreamer' or 'in her own little world' when in fact she may be entirely present but not making the socially required non-verbal signals to indicate that she is. It may be that other senses can be utilized more effectively if a person doesn't have to look at the unfathomable movements of a face at the same time.

> I had a reputation in my family as being someone who did not listen to people. Part of that may have been due to the fact that I often did not look directly at them or did not appear to be attending to them when they spoke to me. They would often say: 'Listen! Use your ears... Look at me when I am speaking to you... Pay attention!'

Some parents observed differences in other non-verbal communication skills that may be typically expected from even a young child, such as pointing and the showing of items. Robyn Steward

(Jansen and Rombout, 2014) says that her mother knew she was autistic when she was only a few months old because she didn't cuddle up to her, make eye contact or point at things. Her mother began to sing to her and that's how they connected with each other.

Once the diagnosis is made, it may be easier to look back and realize what was happening, although at the time with no reference point it would be difficult to pinpoint the root of specific behaviour, such as asking for reassurance to an unusual degree. This could easily be misconstrued as stemming from anxiety, rather than an inability to receive the required data from a face, for example. For clinicians and other professionals, it is important to consider these individual clues through the lens of autism to ascertain their true origin.

> She misses many non-verbal cues and especially struggles with facial expressions and tone of voice and will regularly ask if someone is cross/happy with her as she isn't sure. (Parent)

> I failed middle-school art classes by not being able to match up drawings of faces to emotions. Any faces with open mouths, I labelled as 'in pain' because I associated open mouths with shouting in pain, but they were 'happy', 'surprised', 'amazed'. I read all sad emotions (sadness, lonely, depressed) as boredom and I read anger as constipation because, well, they looked like they were trying really hard to poop.

> I didn't know pointing meant I had to look unless I was explicitly told, and I often couldn't tell what the other person was pointing at. I found it pretty useless myself as a communication tool so didn't really use it.

> There will usually have been some kind of non-verbal or subtle sign that other children do not want her to play, [but] she misses it and the situation escalates. (Parent)

Verbal communication

> I heard the following words and phrases throughout my childhood and adolescence: 'blunt', 'no filter', 'you're so hot and cold', 'you're either 100 per cent or zero', 'there is no in-between with you', 'you are cold' (a.k.a. unfeeling), so 'matter of fact', 'rude' (even when I thought I was being polite).

Language has always been part of the diagnostic criteria for ASDs but was dropped in the latest DSM-5 criteria as a distinct measure. Autistic individuals present a varied profile across language ability, both in speech and language comprehension. Some individuals are entirely non-verbal throughout their lives yet may have good intellect and sophisticated understanding. The majority of those questioned for this book had early speech, advanced vocabulary and sometimes 'incessant chatter'. This was the case even when the general learning profile of the child was delayed or weak in other areas. Speech and language were precocious in many of these girls and something that those around them especially noticed. I was one of these children; my mother reported that I spoke full sentences by the time I was nine months old. It is likely that due to the weight given to verbal ability and speech, as indications of both intelligence and social skill, the eloquence of these girls may have distracted parents and clinicians from considering autism as a potential diagnosis.

Rather than the 'extreme autistic aloneness' personality mentioned by Kanner (1943, p.242), Kopp and Gillberg (1992) saw girls in their study being more 'clinging' (p.96) to others, imitating their speech and movements without a deeper understanding of the unspoken laws of ordinary social interaction. They also saw more repetitive questioning and 'almost constant use of language' (p.97), which is not commonly expected in the typical (male) profile of autism. This verbosity can appear social and interactive, but may be, on examination, scripted, overly formal, learned or largely self-centric in nature.

> Aged three, when she had something in her eye, she said, 'I have an obstruction in my pupil'. (Parent)

> I could speak eloquently by age two. My mother often describes it like I 'swallowed a dictionary' [...] My comprehension of language was always very high though I would use words hollowly; [I knew] the context but not the exact meaning.

This may have caused parents and professionals to overlook potential social difficulties, because speech was profuse and advanced in amount and vocabulary, even though it was not necessarily so adept in pragmatics (Attwood, 2012). In contrast, these girls were also seen to have social difficulties in understanding social cues and reciprocal relationship development, despite their verbosity and apparent sociability.

It is important that speech is not seen as the fundamental measure of intelligence or social skills, as it can be deceptive and misleading for both verbal and non-verbal individuals across the autism spectrum. It is necessary to look beneath the vocabulary and analyse the quality and nature of the communication and relationship dynamics. The words may be scripts learned from a favourite TV show or overheard on a bus; the meaning might not be understood to the level that the eloquent and precise speech might suggest.

> I spoke on time, but used a lot of echolalic speech (e.g. if I hurt myself, I'd say 'Does it hurt?' rather than 'I am hurt'). I also used quite pedantic speech with long words and spoke in very formal language.

> She has difficulty with idiom, sarcasm, tone of voice [and] multiple and complex instructions. This becomes increasingly evident as her peers begin to understand these language usages. It was less obvious when she was younger as very few of the children had these skills. (Parent)

Autistic individuals are often described as 'literal', but this does not always fully encompass what this means in reality. One such resulting behaviour can be a wonderful and brutal bluntness and honesty that often accompany autism at all ages. Many typical children are known to speak their mind and say inappropriate things, but those children will undoubtedly learn from their mistakes and quickly learn the skills of verbal and non-verbal subtlety, which, along with empathy, allow for more gentle interactions. This behaviour can be particularly poorly tolerated in girls, who are expected to be tactful.

> 'Fat grandmothers don't ride bikes.'
> [...] 'Liane, let your grandmother ride your new bike.'
> 'No. She is too fat and she will break it.' [...]
> And off I rode, on my bike, no fat grandmas with me. (Holliday Willey, 2001, p.39)

The resulting reprimand for this type of truthfulness is deeply puzzling for the autistic girl who has yet to learn that sometimes honesty is not the best policy. For one girl, the ability to imagine the emotional consequences of her factually accurate words also led to her being negatively received due to the connotations wrongly applied to her intentions by others.

> We were playing a game in class where you wrote down someone's future on lollipop sticks and put them in a cup. Whatever lollipop stick you picked, that would be your future. I wrote down (for some reason), 'this person will get cancer'... I had no ill-will or negativity for that situation or future prediction. I just thought that it was something that happened – no negative or positivity attached to it.

Autistic individuals can be literal, both in their own speech and in interpreting that of others, in ways that a non-autistic person couldn't possibly predict or appreciate. This difficulty in seeing beyond the actual (literal) meaning of what has been said is a constant cause of anxiety for many on the autism spectrum because it generally involves other people (social interaction) and a potential for failure, confusion or something unexpected happening, all of which are stressful and to be avoided. The examples provided by my women respondents were both brilliant and painful, and beautifully illustrate what a baffling and distressing world they had to endure as small children. I could have presented an entire chapter on these head-scratching encounters.

> When I was about seven I asked my mum how old she was and she told me she was 21 (she was in fact about 50!), but I believed her; and when I told my teacher this and my teacher insisted that she couldn't be 21, I felt betrayed. I had no idea why my mother would lie about such a thing.

> I remember being aware when I was about five that older kids did their 'tables', as in times-tables. I imagined this involved stacking tables on top of each other and was gutted to find out it didn't.

> I was being presented with a perfect attendance award at a school ceremony, and I did not respond several times when my name was called. When my mother asked me why I did not respond when my name was called, I told her that I wasn't sure if there were other XXs in the audience (i.e. others having the same first and last name) and I wasn't sure it was me they were talking about. At that time, I did not know that a person's first name/last name combination was unique to each single person in most instances.

> My mum organized a costume party. I remember that during the party all I wanted to do was to change in and out of costumes, until I had found the right one. The other girls wanted to play, and they kept telling me they were bored. I did not realize that the reason for a costume party was to play as usual, only dressed up. I thought costume parties were to play at changing costumes.

Managing uncertainty

Factors relating to change, focus shifting and unknowns are all part of the autistic profile. In real life, these can reveal themselves in strong preferences for sameness, repetition and needing to know what will happen at all times. The inheritability of autism can be a blessing for some autistic girls growing up in families where similar characteristics may be inherent in parents:

> We had a set routine and saw few new people. We didn't go on holidays or visit new places and did not have birthday parties. I did not have to cope with much change [...] I think my parents were both on the spectrum and liked what was familiar.

The fight-or-flight response to unexpected situations and occurrences is well documented in autism and reported by parents describing their girls' behaviour. Parents can find themselves needing to be alert to potential triggers in order to maintain the safety of their children. Alternatively, parents struggle with a child whose response to an unpredictable world is to avoid it at all costs and remain in the sanctuary of their familiar home. Parents can feel that their daughter 'should' be sociable, and they experience extreme guilt and sadness at her perceived isolation, whereas the child herself feels quite happy, calm and safe at home engaged in her own interests.

> She would prefer to stay at home and never go out, so life is stressful for all of us trying to persuade her to lead a normal life. (Parent)

> We are able to change routines if we do it slowly and give her a good explanation and a long enough presentation period; this is tricky as it is dependent on the situation – if we introduce a change or proposed trip too early, then she has increased anxiety and obsessive questioning! (Parent)

> I sat at the same spot in all my classes in secondary school and college... If it was my seat, it was my seat, and I rarely ever let it go because I would feel very uncomfortable. The seat any farther from or closer to the window would make me feel hotter or colder than I usually am, a seat closer to the door would feel like I'm spilling out of the room. It just felt off and wrong, so it had to be my seat.

Play and toy preference

Choice of play can be one of the earliest indicators of autism (Riley-Hall, 2012). Interestingly, one of the findings from research into sex differences in autistic children was that autistic girls do not have the same stereotypical, rigid interests as boys (Carter *et al.*, 2007). My research certainly found that repetitive and restricted behaviours were completely the norm for the girls studied but that topic type differed. A small number of activities came up time and time again as being favourites for repetition: watching the same TV/video/DVD programme (e.g. *Mary Poppins*, *Postman Pat*, *Peppa Pig*), reading the same book (e.g. an Enid Blyton book, *Jane Eyre*, a Harry Potter book) or listening to the same song/tape. The scripts and lyrics of their favourite shows, books and songs were all known verbatim by the children.

> As an eight-year-old girl, I knew the entire songs and dialogue to the films *Sound of Music*, *Chitty Chitty Bang Bang*, *Annie* and *Mary Poppins*.

Collecting and sorting specific objects were also mentioned. I recall spending many hours attempting to devise an efficient means of systemizing my extensive collection of Lego but was conflicted about the criteria that should be applied – size of block, colour or function – and never succeeded in finding a system that satisfied me. It still disturbs me when contemplating my grandchildren's Lego; they are less concerned. Although this is still the same core behaviour associated with autism, I think that there is a qualitative difference between male 'lining up' behaviour and female behaviour. The girls' activities often involved people and/or animals, rather than objects (aside from an almost universal love of Lego). These people may be fictional characters – real or animated, actors or musicians. The girls' behaviour also all involves words and communication on some level.

> [She] would act out scenarios she had witnessed (real or books or films). The same scenes would be played over and over again [...] She would always include the 'he said' or 'she said' after dialogue – as if she was reading from a book. (Parent)

Given the early and advanced speech mentioned by many interviewed and research (Chellew *et al.*, 2022), there does appear to be – in my sample at least – some desire for communication, language or words by many of these girls at an early age, even if the purpose and intuitive understanding of the social rules are not necessarily present. Surely it is no coincidence that, despite reported numbers of autistic women being significantly lower than those of men, many of the most established and prolific authors in autism – particularly those telling their own story – are women. Perhaps autistic women have an innate drive to communicate.

Knickmeyer, Wheelwright and Baron-Cohen (2008) examined sex-typical play in autistic girls. Their research found that autistic girls did not show a preference for female-typical items when engaged in play that did not involve pretence. This may show evidence of the hypothesis of masculinization in autistic girls; alternatively, the researchers suggest these girls may be less susceptible to social factors that influence toy selection by girls and boys. However, if this were the case, we may have expected them to find the same lack of preference for gender-based non-pretence toys in autistic boys, but this was not the case: boys showed a preference for sex-typical non-pretence toys. When looking at games that did involve pretence (imagination), autistic boys showed virtually no interest, whereas autistic girls were very much engaged in imaginary play, as per typically developing girls. Imagination, usually considered to be an area of difficulty in autistic individuals, may not be affected in the same way in girls as it is in boys, with girls often retreating into fantasy worlds as respite from the stress of being in the real one. The Knickmeyer *et al.* (2008) study also cites research that suggests that pretence may be a skill that is developed via nurture more in girls than in boys: parent–daughter pretence play is more likely than parent–son pretence play.

In those asked, toy preference in girls was overwhelmingly driven towards toys designed for 'doing', rather than imagining or pretending. Knickmeyer *et al.* (2008) found that autistic girls did not show a preference for female-typical items when engaged in play that did not involve pretence. Cars, Lego, construction, Pokémon, robots and monsters all featured. Even for girls who loved having soft, cuddly toys and dolls, the play was more in organizing, collecting and sorting rather than interactive and imaginative play with these items. These toys are often unnamed or given literal names based on specific, factual criteria rather than imaginatively: an orange bear is named 'Orange Bear', a dog with a large nose is named 'Big Nose'.

> I must have been around two years old when my grandmother gave me a doll. I remember how much I disliked it. I put it in the bin.

The autistic girl may have more dolls than her peers, but these may be arranged in a specific order and not used for shared imaginative play (Attwood *et al.*, 2006). For those girls who did play out scenarios with teddies and dolls, it is generally anecdotally reported by parents and individuals to often be verbatim scripts of earlier events or replications of parental behaviours. One child would re-enact her school day word for word with her toys at home (this was verified by the parent asking the teacher about the day). On first appearance, these activities can look very typical and imaginative, but this may not always be the true picture. A child who talks to herself out loud and puts on different voices may not be creating imaginary characters and complex worlds, but may be repeating TV shows, conversations and events that she has actually experienced. It is important that accurate and detailed information about the content of the play is gathered, as taking the observation at face value may be misleading.

> When she does play with girls' toys, she has very prescriptive play – undresses them all and puts them all to bed – with no story or interaction between dolls. (Parent)

> [...]Gave my soft toys idiosyncratic or functional names – Best Ted, Fat Ted ('Fat' used in a descriptive rather than a derogatory sense).

Some girls in my sample didn't play with any toys at all, preferring to be outside, active and enjoying nature. Tony Attwood includes an interest in nature in his girls' screening questionnaire (GQ-ASC) (Attwood 2013).

> I did not play with the typical toys; I preferred to be outside running free.

Other commonly reported activities included colouring, collecting items and reading. Many autistic girls are self-taught readers (Simone, 2010), learning quickly and voraciously devouring any book they can find, whether information-based or fiction. As Rudy Simone says: 'Information replaces confusion' (Simone, 2010, p.23). Not only does reading offer a solo escape from a chaotic world; it also provides knowledge and data that may help the girl to manage that world once she has to return to it. Shared pretend play didn't appeal to many of the girls in my survey; they preferred to be 'doing' rather than 'being', unless, that is, they were immersed in a solo fantasy world of their own creation; more about that in a moment.

Encouraging interests and desire for knowledge is a good way to support and motivate an autistic girl. Parents and professionals may be concerned about her isolation and lack of social interaction, but it may be that school or family life overwhelms her far more quickly than it does other children, and allowances need to be made for her to be alone in order to replenish her capacity. If this is not appreciated, eventual shutdown, meltdown and/or increased anxiety will be the almost inevitable result.

> She loves books and plays with them as well as reading them – almost like they have their own personalities. (Parent)

Play was almost exclusively solo for the girls in my sample under the age of around six years, although some girls did seek out the company of others but found that it only took a very short time for them to either offend the other children or become upset with the notion of shared play. The girl appears to take either a domineering role, in which all activities have to be on her terms, or a more passive role where she is 'mothered' by more socially able girls. These findings back up another study mentioned earlier (Knickmeyer *et al.*, 2008) that found that girls did not show a preference for 'female-typical' items in non-pretence play, whereas autistic boys did show a preference for 'male-typical' items. In pretend play, autistic girls show a preference for same-sex-typical toys (as do autistic boys). One suggestion is that autistic girls are more likely to have learned how to do pretend play from their parents, as this is often more encouraged in girls than in boys. Girls, as we have heard, also appear to be motivated to learn how to fit in and behave as expected of a typical girl, and this may demonstrate a high capability for imitation.

For the few girls who did play with dolls and more traditional female toys, in most cases parents and individuals reported that this appeared to be more from an awareness of what was acceptable and required by other girls in order to be considered for social interaction and friendship.

> My daughter likes pink and princesses. I think this is because the other girls like them – she doesn't actually play with her princess dolls unless her friends are playing with them. She much prefers to be outside collecting flowers and insects. (Parent)

Intense interests

> I developed an interest in *Coronation Street*. Now, it is quite typical to enjoy soap operas, and I knew that it was perfectly okay for me to ask my classmates if they had watched the previous evening's episode. I knew it wasn't perfectly okay for me to tell them how many bricks the Rovers Return was made out of or the exact dates each character had made their first appearance, [or] how I was making a scale model of the set. (Mason, in Hurley, 2014, p.14)

Enjoying an intense interest in one or more subjects is a core element in the profile of autism and is a defining feature of many autistic women's identities (Bargiela *et al.*, 2016) but differences in the specifics of this profile are noted between boys and girls (Attwood, 2012). Boys' interests tend to be object-based – trains, dinosaurs, space – while girls' interests are often focused on people or animals – soap operas, fictional characters and celebrities. This qualitative difference can explain why girls' behaviour may not be noted as being unusual, due to the 'typical girl' nature of their interests (Simone, 2010; Wagner, 2006). Whereas a boy who quotes endless facts about ancient history, rather than playing football with his peers, may be flagged as atypical, a girl who obsesses about a pop star would not necessarily be seen in the same way. The difference between the interests of an autistic girl and a typical child is the narrowness of the topic and the intensity of the interest. These autistic girls have single-track focus; they do not think or speak of anything other than their passion for an extended period. They may have extensive knowledge of their subject but have more of a factual interest than a desire to live it out. A child who speaks of nothing but horses may not actually want a horse, but just enjoys the facts about horses. I believe that the interest provides the same outcomes for both girls and boys on the autism spectrum: once immersed in your subject of interest, there is a predictability and escape from the chaotic real world. Knowing everything about a subject makes it 'known' and provides a sanctuary from the anxiety and stress of a feeling of not knowing what's going to happen most of the time.

Crafting and making things comes up frequently for autistic girls and women as lifelong interests. Often these are 'serial crafters' who move from one medium to another with equal all-consuming passion. As children, this appears to be more of a general desire to 'do' something productive and useful, which then in adulthood can move into a career or a range of specific passions - once finances and time are in one's own control. In early years, the girls like to bake, sew, draw and a whole range of other practical pursuits, which do not require a large amount of imagination. There may be instructions to follow and a fixed outcome to aim for with no pretending required. Logic, function, purpose and practicality will continue to be a strong force throughout their lives from this early point.

Animals are a popular interest as they are far easier to deal with than people for many autistic females: their intentions are clear (no hidden agendas), their non-verbal language is minimal (cats don't pull too many facial expressions), their needs are easily identified and their attachment and affection are unconditional and unchanging. Some girls identify so strongly with animals that they imagine or wish themselves to be one (Attwood, 2007). This, combined with a drive to learn factual information about hammerhead sharks or every known dog breed, makes for a perfect intense enthusiasm to be shared with anyone who will listen, and even those who won't.

> I was a pony before I had one. I cantered everywhere, neighed out loud and jumped imaginary obstacles.

I would suggest that animals are more of a favourite interest for girls than for autistic boys. As previously mentioned, there does seem to be a desire for many of these girls to connect in some way with living beings (people, animals, insects) rather than just with inanimate objects, as the boys tend to do. The nature of this connection, however, may be significantly different than that experienced by typical children.

Typical interests of a girl on the autistic spectrum include:

- anime
- craft
- animals – cats, horses
- nature
- soft toys
- characters from books
- collecting
- TV programmes
- TV/movie actors
- historical characters.

> I collected lots of items, from key rings to daddy long-legs (crane fly) [...] I had an old jar that I filled to bursting with these insects; really awful when I think back to these creatures suffering. I loved to look at them in the jar; I was fascinated with them moving about crammed together.

> She gets fixated with certain people who she admires. These can be real (e.g. an older girl at school), historical (e.g. Princess Vicky, daughter of Queen Victoria) or imagined (e.g. a character from a book or film). (Parent)

> After reading ***The Hobbit*** and ***Lord of the Rings***, she learned the two languages – Quenya and Elvish – and spent hours writing them.
>
> Dinosaurs: age 3–6 approx. Read lots of books on dinosaurs; we visited dinosaur adventure parks; she had lots of dinosaur figures; we went to the Natural History Museum. Also she was late being toilet trained and success was only achieved as a result of dinosaur transfers on knickers and dinosaur progress reward

> sticker charts leading to a visit to the Natural History Museum. She knew more about dinosaurs than the Year 1 teacher.
>
> Cats: age 7–11 approx. Most drawings were of cats. Read all the Warrior Cat books and cat-related books. Most stories and work at school involved cats even when they were irrelevant to the topic. She meowed when the teacher took the register. (We got a cat when she was 6.)
>
> Writing books: 11–14. She would spend hours writing books. When younger she would decide in advance what all the chapters were going to be called, which we found very amusing. Her stories tended to be totally weird and involve characters from other stories, people she knew, YouTubers, etc. (Parent)

Sensory experience

Observable sensory differences can present themselves early on for children on the autism spectrum, and these are likely to be made known in no uncertain terms by an infant or small child. Refusal, screaming and general extreme distress when encountering specific objects or sensations may be an indicator of an inability to tolerate something.

> [She] has an intense dislike of clothes [...] [she] will take them off as soon as she walks through the door and in any household where she knows she can. (Parent)

> I like things to be tight around my waist and not tight around my neck. I hate socks and tend to wear them inside out to get the horrid stitching feeling away from my nails.

> I've had an aversion to water since childhood: being bathed, washing my hair, dishes, touching wet towels, touching small puddles of water on the floor or table, anything that has to do with wetness.

> Headphones are used at school and clothes labels are cut out

> and sensory tights are worn. Visuals are used to help with temperature showing the right clothing for weather. Food is kept to safe food and brands we know she will trust. A chewy necklace is used to help with wanting to bite clothes and nails. And fidget toys for on the way home help keep her busy so [she is] not likely to stop and touch everything (Parent).

> In boarding school, I used to lock myself in the clothes locker. I would open the room window or turn the air conditioning on so the room was cool, set up my blanket inside my locker, remove any item of clothing that was perfumed, put on sleeping ear plugs and close myself in because I needed to be in a cool, dark, quiet place and have as few senses as physically possible.

Equally, for those who discover a sensory experience that soothes and calms, a seeking-out and incessant desire for that stimulus might be noted. Some of these behaviours originate from external sensory stimuli such as noise or tactile textures, while others are self-generated and found to be either enjoyable in their own right or are used as a self-soothing strategy or means of communication in times of stress.

> My number-one preferred activity as a toddler and young child, was rocking, including rocking on my duck, rocking on my rocking horse, rocking on my bed or rocking on the floor.

> She seeks out flashing fairy lights and likes to look at water moving and shadows on the pavement. (Parent)

> Fuzzy things. Any dolls that had hair, furry/fuzzy teddies, and especially my aunt's hot-water-bottle fur case that I stuffed with socks. Also, my sister's hair. She let me play with her hair and I did that so much. I taught myself how to braid with her hair. I still have to stop myself from playing with people's hair if they are sat in front of me, and I still like soft, fuzzy things.

> She seeks out all different textures and will stop on her way home to feel the ground, e.g. stones, leaves, feathers and flowers. (Parent)

> I preferred jogging bottoms and sweatshirts as they were made of soft, smooth, slightly stretchy fabric. Wool clothes physically hurt me, and non-stretchy clothes felt stifling, no matter what their size.

> She seeks water and will spend hours in the bath even when it goes cold. In summer she won't get out of the paddling pool even to eat or drink unless reminded. (Parent)

Liane Holliday Willey (2014) describes how many noises and bright lights made her life unbearable and how she found relief underwater in her 'safety zone' (p.28). Most of the women and parents I questioned list a considerable number of sensory preferences notable from infancy. For those writing as late-diagnosed adults, we cannot always know what these behaviours were attributed to (if anything) when these women were children, but the frequency and severity of some of the behaviours make it difficult to believe that they were not noticed at the time.

> We have many photos of her squishing her face into mesh fabrics, rolling naked in fleece materials, drinking mud from a trowel! (Parent)

> She used to like to push her forehead against the drum of the washing machine on full cycle to feel the vibrations, and would put paper bags on her head as a toddler and just run until she crashed into things. (Parent)

> She has a stereotypical whole-body tic when excited which involves opening and closing her hands while twisting the wrists, curling and flexing her feet and opening her mouth all at the same time. (Parent)

Sharing

> I just did my own thing, and if someone initiated conversation or wanted to play, I'd say something like, 'Sure, I'm playing with this toy, so you can play with that one'.

The notion of sharing is not always one that young children understand: 'Why would I want to give you something that leaves me with less?' The development of theory of mind at around four to six years of age usually changes this perspective and leads the child to understand that if I give you something of mine, there may be a deal here in which I can get something better in return. It is thought that autistic children develop this skill later and sometimes not to the same degree. Needing the world to be 'on their terms' is a common comment made by those living with and supporting autistic individuals. It can appear that the child is extremely self-focused, when it may be that the concept of the needs of others is simply not developed yet. This is a trait less easily tolerated in girls, who are expected to be more intuitive to the needs of others.

Sharing involves:

- change of plan/status quo: 'I was doing this, now I have to adapt'
- other people: 'I have no idea what they might want. It's easier to be on my own'
- non-verbal communication: 'Does this person have a hidden agenda?'
- unpredictability: 'When will I get it back? When will it be my turn?'
- verbal negotiation: On-the-spot, socially acceptable response required
- anticipating the behaviour of another person
- sharing possessions and space: risk, loss of control and safety

- having to do something that you may not want to do.

It is not difficult to see why this doesn't seem like a worthwhile deal at a young age and why solo play is a more logical and low-stress choice for many autistic children. Issues with the concept of sharing were mentioned by a significant number of participants. Some did not necessarily object to it when the consequences and benefits were explained; they simply had not been aware that there was an expectation from others that it should be done.

> She finds sharing very difficult and wants everything to be done on her terms [...] 'Precious' toys have to be hidden away before other children come to play. She would never think to offer sweets to others and refuses to do so when prompted.

> I was capable of sharing and did do it; I just didn't especially want to and didn't understand why the school didn't make adequate provision to ensure that we didn't have to share. It seemed illogical.

Fantasy worlds

One of the common anecdotally reported differences between the male and female presentation of autism concerns the concept of imaginative play, as discussed above. Traditionally, autistic children are considered to not engage in imaginary play due to a limited ability to generate fictional worlds and ideas. The observation of play is normally part of the diagnostic assessment, and the classic lining-up of cars that many people associate with autism is thought to be a clear indicator of differences or limits in the typically expected imagination. In girls, however, something different is sometimes seen, which may seem contradictory to the comments presented above that stated that girls were less creative in their games. Individually and privately, autistic girls are known to sometimes inhabit a rich fantasy world full of imaginary friends, animals and creatures (Attwood, 2007; Holliday Willey, 2014). Having imaginary friends is not particularly unusual for any child, but as Tony Attwood (2007) says, 'the child with Asperger's syndrome [*sic*] may *only* have friends who are imaginary, and the intensity and duration of the imaginary interactions can be qualitatively unusual' (p.25).

> I much preferred the company of my imaginary friends. Penny and her brother Johnna were my best friends, though no one saw them but me. My mother tells me I used to insist that we set them places at the table, include them on our car trips, and treat them like they were real beings. (Holliday Willey, 2014, p.19)

> The biggest universe I ever created originally contained about 100 creatures, but this is now over 1000, as this universe has stuck with me throughout my entire life [...] This fantasy is a place I would often slip into as a child, especially when I wished to avoid other people. I had in excess of 64 imaginary friends, and I much preferred playing with these characters than interacting with anyone at all.

I believe that this is not a contradiction but represents a difference in what autistic girls present visibly in terms of play and games (often when others are involved), and what really goes on in their private worlds inside their heads where there are no boundaries, restrictions or social rules. Having no interest in fiction is an indicator on some autism assessment tools that were developed through investigation of the male profile (due to larger numbers of males available for sampling, rather than any deliberate intent to exclude females). However, overwhelmingly what we see in girls is an unusually extreme identification with the characters in fiction books, TV programmes and sometimes people they know and feel an attachment to: the girls actually 'become' the character. This may involve re-enacting scenes from the book, film or show over and over again, mimicry, and getting lost in the fantasy to the point of having difficulty in separating it from real life. As mentioned previously, we also see girls who identify far more closely with animals than humans and believe and behave as though they are a cat, for example. One young woman, aged 18, whom I worked with, said that she didn't want to grow up as adulthood seemed too scary, and that if she were a cat, people would take care of her. She would often wear a tail and cat ears.

> She was obsessed with Postman Pat's cat, Jess, and would like to be talked to as a cat and reply in cat language. (Parent)

From a diagnostic perspective, it is possible that this could be viewed as delusion or psychosis, whereas for the girls I spoke to, it was more of an escape to a better place from a real world that was difficult and sometimes unhappy.

> I used to disappear to some local hilly fields and roam around pretending I was Maria, from *The Sound of Music*, singing my head off. Fantasy was my escape. In my pretend world, I was an amazing, talented girl.

> I much preferred my imaginary world to reality and would spend as much time as I could (apart from when I was reading) thinking about my fantasy world. I often hated getting out of bed because that was a great place to think about my imaginary friends undisturbed, and having to drag myself away from that and return to reality was horrible and depressing.

Clothing

Universally, for those responding there was a strong preference for clothing that was comfortable, soft, stretchy, loose and smooth. For many, there was also a distinct dislike of clothes that the child considered to be 'girly' (their word). So, not only is there a sensory preference or dislike regarding certain textures, colours or fabrics, but also an active choice around types of clothing (skirts, dresses) typically associated with girls. Kopp and Gillberg (2011) report 'careless with physical appearance' as a feature specific to autistic girls. I would question the use of the word 'careless' in this assessment, which is an external, observational judgement.

The individual themselves may have taken great care in avoiding certain clothing or textures – the results may look 'careless' or atypical but may be anything but. It could be suggested that clothing choice in this form may also illustrate something about gender identity and social conformity at an early age in these girls, a subject that will be discussed in greater detail later. Certainly, these girls and women were not generally likely to suffer discomfort in the name of fashion (which is surely a measure of social awareness).

Toileting and personal hygiene

Toileting issues are commonly reported in autistic individuals, so this should not come as a surprise: social rules, sensory issues and unpredictability are all involved in toileting and personal hygiene. The causes may be varied, but anxiety and irritable bowel syndrome are well documented anecdotally as issues for autistic individuals, and it is possible that this could make it harder for a child to keep themselves clean. Obviously, it is important to rule out physical causes for toileting difficulties before making assumptions that they are psychological.

> I didn't use the toilet completely independently until I was around 11 as I needed help to wipe my behind on defecating. I eventually learned to do this myself but had problems with what I now know to be irritable bowel syndrome my entire life, including childhood.

> Late to train, but because of extreme fear of poo not her inability to hold and use the toilet. It took ages for her to wipe herself, through worry of poo; she used baby wipes at first and then moved on to toilet roll. (Parent)

> When I was two or three, I had a special toilet seat and would not go to the toilet unless it was on that special seat.

> I wet my bed until I was 15 years old. (Jansen and Rombout, 2014, p.99)

Participants cited difficulties with recognizing the physical signals that indicated a need to go to the toilet, as well as anxiety around using toilet facilities outside their own homes. An expectation that toilet and hygiene rules and behaviour would be intuitive was reported by some women, who were aware that they had 'got this wrong' because the context of why these things were important (and how to do them properly) was assumed to be understood and therefore not taught.

> I was punished severely for not cleaning myself properly [...] If only they had just shown me how to do it properly.

Adolescent characteristics

> The teenage years were the worst years of my life. I was clueless to the world and felt like a fish out of water. Puberty and body changes were embarrassing and 'yuk' too.

Where do I begin?! Take a socially awkward, quiet tomboy who doesn't relate to her female peers, and throw a load of hormones at her. That's not going to go down well!

Puberty and adolescence are frequently a difficult time for all young women, but the combination of adolescence and autism brings its own set of challenges. Families talk about not knowing from one day to the next whether the young person's behaviour can be best explained by autism or their age (Nichols *et al.*, 2009). Friendships change, expectations change, bodies change and feelings change (that's if you can work out what you are feeling at all). It's a lot to handle for someone who takes a while to get used to change, especially when she may not be ready for these changes and just wants to carry on building Lego and pretending to be a pony (meanwhile her classmates are swooning over some pop star and obsessing over what to wear).

> At some point in sixth grade (when I was about 11), many of the

> girls in my class became huggers. They hugged when they met each other and when they said goodbye. They hugged when they passed in the hallway. They hugged when they were happy or sad. They hugged and cried and squealed with excitement and I watched from a distance, perplexed. What did all this hugging mean? And more importantly, why wasn't I suddenly feeling the need to hug someone every 30 seconds? (Kim, in Hurley, 2014, p.24)

On the whole, women in my survey who had been through adolescence, often without a diagnosis of autism, did not have a good word to say about this time in their lives. A few reported positively, but they were often those who had successfully located a like-minded oddball or a kind neurotypical pal who gave them the acceptance that they were desperate to find; alternatively, they were the type of girl who was able to live quite happily without that acceptance. Women were asked to describe their teenage years, and the following examples are typical of the emotions remembered:

> [...] Locked in. Caged and ultimately restricted. It's a period of my life that is a relative blur since it was so uneventful, when for most people it's a monumental time of self-discovery, exploration of the world at large and forging new directives in the way of career and life perspective, etc.

> I struggled to cope with public transport and used to walk the two miles each way to school rather than get the bus. I don't know why I found it difficult – probably just the compulsory interaction with the bus driver and my peers on the bus. I just couldn't cope with it. I was allowed so little time alone that the 40-minute walk to school and back, alone, was a relief.

Some of the typical diagnostic characteristics of ASD can be less obvious as a girl gets older – this may particularly apply to more intellectually able and self-aware individuals who learn what is required and what is deemed unacceptable. Young autistic women, as we have heard, are often excellent social anthropologists, studying the behaviours of others in order to predict more accurately what neurotypicals will do, and also to imitate this behaviour themselves in order to receive either social approval or, at the very least, slip under the radar to some degree. Despite their best efforts, it is often the case that their female peers are not fooled and that some aspects of their autistic profile remain visible to others.

> Socially, I suspect I came across as cold and aloof to people, which is a shame as I'm not like that, but I don't pull the faces and do the gestures that NTs are so taken with, so I am judged negatively before people even bother to get to know me.

> My teens were full of 'what you f**king looking at?' by other girls. This was incredibly confusing and frightening to me. Obviously, something in my facial expression was upsetting them, but I really don't know what.

Intense interests exist throughout the lifetime of autistic people, but they can change and develop with age. For young women in my sample, reading still featured heavily, as it had done when they were children. Drawing, writing, sewing and collecting were all reported – these productive activities often remain with them throughout adulthood as they become serial crafters and which may even become a career. The interests mentioned are solitary pursuits and no one mentioned sharing these interests with peers (other than video-gaming, which was remote interaction rather than in the same room). People still formed a significant part of the young women's interests, either through fictional characters or obsessions or crushes on people known to them. The solitary nature of these interests could lead to the assumption of shyness, isolation, depression or social anxiety – all of which may be the case, but which, equally, may mask underlying autism.

> I was into music big time. I preferred music from before my day and disliked the stuff my peers were into. During my teens I liked

> rock and roll music from the 50s and 60s and would play my favourite tracks over and over again; I knew all the words and all about the artists.

> In my teens I was obsessed with the Royal Navy. Then I think my obsessions were mostly people – partners and the future I hoped to build with them. I also spent several years obsessed by cricket, both playing and watching.

> I have spent much of my teenage and adult years reading fiction, playing computer games and watching fiction on TV. Many times I've felt closer to fictional characters than real-life people.

Puberty and hygiene

Understanding and knowledge about matters involving physical and hormonal changes during puberty may be more limited in this group of girls due to their potentially limited peer group, which is typically the main source of this information for most young people. Support to ensure that young autistic women receive this information and have the opportunity to ask questions is essential. Shana Nichols *et al.* (2009) have written *Girls Growing Up on the Autism Spectrum,* a comprehensive guide to supporting girls in dealing with all issues relating to puberty and adolescence. Witnessing your own body changing without any understanding of what is happening can lead to anxiety and fear about something that is perfectly normal. An autistic girl may not feel able to talk to anyone about her worries as she may be afraid that there is something wrong with her.

> At about the age of 11, I found a magazine in the newsagents called the *Mizz Book of Love*. This magazine was a treasure trove of factual info about puberty, sex, STI [sexually transmitted infection], pregnancy, etc. Thank God I found this magazine. I was not shocked at puberty because I knew what to expect; in fact, I was excited and happy to change into a woman. I am

> certain that educating young girls on the spectrum in depth is essential. I already discuss the facts of life, including sex abuse, with my six-year-old daughter – she can ask me anything and I will tell her. I feel very strongly about this. She needs to know.

Some young women don't know when they should start to wear a bra or how to have that conversation with their parents or carers. Wearing a bra takes some getting used to, particularly if you have sensory sensitivity to touch. It can be unbearably uncomfortable. Nichols *et al.* (2009) discuss the issue of bras and how to address the concept. Some autistic women continue into adulthood choosing not to wear a bra, which is a personal right but one that comes with potential consequences. I worked with a young woman with very large breasts who did not see why she should wear a bra but was not aware that her bosom was very obvious and that people stared at her and made negative comments. Her decision may also have had implications for her physical health as she had no support for her breasts and her back. The decision was hers to make, but she needed to have honest advice about other people's perceptions and any health implications in order to enable her to make an informed choice. She continued to not wear a bra as she didn't care what people thought. Some autistic women do not wish to conform to societal norms that they feel do not fit them and should be supported to do so once they know all the consequences.

Hygiene is another area that takes on greater importance from the onset of puberty, with some young autistic women not really understanding or being concerned about the health and social impacts of being dirty and smelling bad. The consequences and actual skills of self-care may need to be taught in detail. It cannot be assumed that the autistic individual knows how much shampoo to use and how to rinse it out, and what the purpose of deodorant is. Parents of autistic teenage girls report that they continue to have a 'hands-on' role with their daughters' hygiene as the girls struggle to be independent and consider what needs doing and why (Cridland *et al.*, 2014).

> I have to remind her to shower every day... And she'll get in the shower, and she'll stand there and play with the water if I don't remind her to put her shampoo in her hair and rinse it... After years of having showers and baths she's not bothering to learn and yet she can learn really complicated things. (Cridland *et al.*, 2014, p.1268)

> Keeping up with hygiene has been one of the hardest things to learn to get used to from childhood to adulthood. My caretakers recall me fighting to get bathed or have my teeth brushed or get my hair brushed. I hate getting wet, so showering requires a lot of self-talk; toothbrushes hurt, and toothpaste burns so brushing my teeth requires a lot of self-talk.

> [...] Still not great with personal hygiene; I mostly wash in order to stop getting sore or so that other people don't think I'm stinky. Being stinky doesn't really worry me.

> I didn't really understand the purpose of personal hygiene. When I started boarding, aged eight, some of the other girls noticed I didn't clean my teeth, so I became more self-aware of things like this. I still only clean my teeth when I'm going to see other people or if it's been about three days since I last brushed and they feel dirty.

In summary

Overall, we can conclude that the teenage years are a time of enormous change, development and learning for young autistic women. All young people find these years difficult at times but the social exclusion and changing nature of friendships, along with increased expectations from families and teachers, mean that young autistic women are faced with additional challenges.

Chapter 4

ADULTHOOD

> *My favourite way to think of autism is this: I miss what others catch, and I catch what others miss.*
>
> Kotowicz (2022, p.19)

> *As years go by, you get better and better at camouflaging and compensating for the external behavioural characteristics of autism. You make the impression of functioning normally by cognitively compensating for what you do not sense or know intuitively due to your autistic way of thinking.*
>
> Jansen and Rombout (2014, p.23)

As adolescence passes and adulthood ensues, expectations and requirements change, but being autistic in a world where most people are not remains. With most research and support firmly focused on autistic children, adults plough on regardless. For our women, many of whom have spent their childhood and teenage years learning how to mask their difficulties and hide and slip under the radar of weirdness, adulthood is merely a continuation of that facade along with a whole set of new and increased requirements to be independent, navigate the adult world and perhaps earn a wage. But...adulthood also brings new autonomy and, with it, the ability to make choices about where, how and with whom we can live, all of which were not available in earlier years when other people made those choices on our behalf.

The majority of these women are getting through each day with an often-sophisticated set of compensatory behaviours, personas and clever strategies to permit them to hide in plain sight and not receive unwanted negative attention. Their ability to do this is testament to an extraordinary resilience and sometimes stubborn determination not to 'fail' or be 'outed' as a 'weirdo'. Unfortunately, these efforts can come at a price: exhaustion, breakdown and other mental health issues are commonly mentioned by these women. These ill-effects are the consequences of living as an autistic person, not conditions or symptoms to be considered in isolation. This is an important point that clinicians must address. Being autistic in a non-autistic world can break a person – and often more than once as those who experience autistic burnout can testify.

The symptoms of the breakage are not the issues to be treated or addressed; the difficulty of living in a non-autistic world as an autistic person is the key. We will look at health implications a little later on. This chapter will focus on the core characteristics of autism that adult women report as having an impact on their lives. I also wanted to know what the women loved about being autistic. Traits that the women liked in themselves were focused on their determination and ability to challenge themselves in difficult times.

> Being independent, learning to cope with adversity, being determined when I want to learn something new, being good at trying things such as DIY so I have become quite good at it. I am very arty and possibly having AS [Asperger syndrome] has helped with that. I am honest, too, and caring and thoughtful.

> I love my sense of duty, my sense of rightness and justice, and my honesty. I will return change to a shop because it is *wrong* to keep it if it isn't mine. My passion for reading means I have specialist knowledge on very niche subjects, and I enjoy that.

> Ability to become immersed in secondary (fantasy) worlds. Sense of the ridiculous and unusual humour (probably seen sometimes by others as childishness). Understanding and communication

> with animals and appreciation of the natural world. Having an analytical mind. Intense focus and attention to detail. Being different and being unique. Sense of morality and opposition to injustice. Being trustworthy and dependable.

Adult indicators

When considering the characteristics of autism that manifest most significantly for these adult women, we must continue to bear in mind societal expectations for women. For example, you will read quotes from women below who hate to share their things; this is not acceptable behaviour for an adult woman who is supposed to be sharing and caring. While some of these characteristics may be equally applicable to other genders of autistic people, the gender expectation factor for females may increase the negative response to these traits from others (which therefore increases the impact on self-esteem and consequently mental health).

All of the diagnostic criteria for autism remain relevant for adult autistic women but these are experienced differently as an adult – as one might expect given that no adult is the same as they were as a child, regardless of the presence of autism (although that doesn't stop some people commenting that: 'You can't be autistic, you are nothing like my seven-year-old autistic nephew'!).

Non-verbal communication

> I am so consumed with how other people are feeling, probably because I spent so many years operating under the assumption that everything I did was 'wrong' or 'bad'. So I think I'm hyper-attuned to how other people might react. Now, I have *no idea* if I'm right or not, that's the problem. Sometimes I assume someone's mad at me, and when I bring it up they act like I'm crazy or imagining things. I definitely have a hard time correctly identifying people's feelings, but it's not for lack of trying.

As mentioned above, adult autistic women have often learned that facial expressions, body language and eye contact are required if one wishes to fit into the neurotypical (NT) world without remonstration, and they have become rather good at presenting themselves in a manner that does not attract attention. They are often keenly aware of how they have constructed a means of minimizing discomfort while maximizing invisibility and social inclusion. These women start out as 'little psychologists' and by adulthood can be masters at analysing social behaviour and emulating it. It must be noted that this is usually not intuitive: it involves conscious awareness and effort 100 per cent of the time while in any social environment, which is draining.

> It's very draining trying to figure out everything all the time: everything is more like on a manual; you've got to use one of those computers where you have to type every command in. (Bargiela *et al.*, 2016, p.3287)

> Until about 13/14 years of age, all body language to me was 'bothered', 'unbothered', 'suspicious' or 'too close to me / in my bubble'.

> I do eye contact, but I'm a mouth reader. Eye contact is completely distracting for me although I have learned that if you look in between the eyes, the other person will think you are doing the whole eyeball thing.

> I was around 50 years old when I realized that people were making eye contact with me when we are speaking socially (as opposed to when I gave a presentation – then I knew they were looking at me). Since then, I work at making eye contact with people. I have no idea what I was doing before.

> I am physically incapable of looking in someone's face or eyes, I just don't see the point because I get uncomfortable being in an intense staring match with someone. I don't know when to blink,

> I don't know which eyeball to look at; I get distracted noticing the pattern of their iris and zits and other facial features I never noticed before.

Even those who do not find masking their differences easy show an incredible awareness of what they 'get wrong' and how they compensate, despite having no means (and in some cases, no desire) of fixing it and doing otherwise.

> [...] Intense eye contact once obtained (staring sternly), [I] rated people's intent purely on the basis of voice, being capable of understanding only the most apparent facial expressions (but would have trouble telling if, say, a smile was a genuine smile and not just a strained one even then). I still rely on intonation to tell me what I need to know about a person's emotions.

And it is not only the reading of non-verbal social gestures from others that is notable for autistic women; having a flat facial affect, that is, not making socially typical facial expressions, is a long-standing autistic characteristic. There's even a name for it in these modern times: 'resting bitch face'! Autistic women are often accidental queens of RBF where their internal mood does not match their external expression.

> As an adult, people often ask if I am okay. I really don't know what my face is saying.

> I was once at a company event where an artist walked around drawing people's faces. I was so excited, but when I got mine, I looked like I was angry. I remember a man being there when I received mine, and he said, 'That's you!' I was shocked to hear that I looked angry all the time.

These last comments remind me of a situation where I was being photographed for a magazine article. I thought I was giving the photographer my best smile, but then he said, 'You look like you want to kill me'. This was a major revelation at the age of 42 when I realized that what I thought I was expressing on my face was nothing like the reality. It explained why 'smile, it might never happen' has been a common and, up until now, bemusing, comment from complete strangers throughout my life. This prompted me to spend several hours looking in a mirror and I realized that my face doesn't move anywhere near as much as I thought it did. Practising facial expressions is a fairly common behaviour reported by autistic women to overcome this.

> Through lots of trial and error, I learned which facial muscles on my face match which expressions in a photo. Now, a posed photo of me looks almost as good as a candidly captured moment of joy. (Kotowicz, 2022, p.46)

Verbal communication

> I've been told I'm very blunt and direct, and I often offend people without meaning to. Apparently I come across as aggressive. I like to get to the point of something, and all the superfluous detail irritates me.

Autistic women tend to be either direct, straightforward and blunt in their communication style – most of us have heard someone say: 'You can't say that!' many times in our lives – or extremely cautious, silent and monitoring their social performance constantly for fear of making a *faux pas*. Both of these opposing presentations occur as a result of having difficulties picking up the subtleties of non-verbal cues, which are generally accepted as necessary and intuitive in the non-autistic world. The blunt approach is often considered not typical for a female and received not only very negatively, but also with an incorrect assumption that it was intentional. The woman herself is frequently bemused as to why she has caused such a response, since from her perspective she was only stating the truth or asking directly for the clarity she needed. Previously, it was suggested that autistic girls are treated less favourably than boys when it comes to perceived rudeness, and this does not abate in adulthood. Many autistic women prefer the company of men and/or other autistic people because they feel less judged for what they see as simply their straightforward communication – saying it like it is. It is also easier to understand what others are saying if it is without nuance and hidden agenda. Autistic women often mention their confusion about why people ask questions that they don't actually want the honest answer to. 'Does my bum look big in this?' and other emotionally loaded questions require a multitude of cognitive skills that autistic women can find hard to muster in the split-second before a response is required – wait too long to reply and the silence speaks volumes. Fortunately, through trial and error, our autistic women have learned that the right answer to this question is always 'No', regardless of the actual truth.

With regard to engaging in superficial small talk, adult autistic women generally don't like it or 'get it'. Difficulties with non-verbal cues can also result in interrupting and missing the flow of conversation. This, combined with a preference for talking about oneself and one's own interests, all add up to someone whose conversation style is not always appreciated. The effort involved in consciously trying to work out what to say or do in the midst of a fast-moving conversation explains the short time capacity for people interactions that many autistic women describe.

> Social occasions involve a more elaborate flowchart. It starts with 'Hello' and, depending on the response, goes into a series of fixed scripts from there.

> Once a colleague started asking me a detailed question without any context. I wish I'd said, 'Sorry, I need some background info first. Can you please explain the purpose of what you're trying to do?' Instead, I curtly replied 'Wait – back up – context'. (Kotowicz, 2022, p.31)

> I still have issues with turn-taking in conversation. If I don't say

> something the second I think of it, then it is lost – often forever – so I interrupt a lot and talk over people. I'd say I'm more aware of when I'm interrupting than I used to be and better at reining myself in when necessary.

> I can be very self-centred. These days I have to make a conscious effort to pretend to be interested in how somebody else is so I can be considered nice, but really all I want to do is talk about myself.

> When I am feeling tired, my ability to process words becomes incredibly diminished. I feel sheer exhaustion just having to listen to people. In times like this, I also lose the ability to speak properly and can end up slurring or forgetting words completely.

> I wrote notes and letters to people instead of trying to a have a conversation verbally. I would also let my close friends read pages from my diary if I wanted to let them know how I was feeling, then I would ask them if they got it, and the conversation would be done without me adding any more information, because I felt like what I had written [had] said what I wanted them to know in the best way I could say it... I would just sit in silence not really expecting questions or verbal confirmation or validation.

The result of these communication differences can be that autistic women misunderstand the words of others as well as being misunderstood themselves. Jokes, sarcasm and a tendency to take things literally can cause confusion, anxiety and a general feeling of stupidity at not having 'got it'. This is not to say that autistic women do not have a sense of humour – they may be quick-witted with their own jokes – but the jokes of others may be lost on them at times (perhaps it's just that the jokes of others are not funny). I have been told on more than one occasion that I can't be autistic because I have a sense of humour and know how to tell a joke. While this is true, I am still unable to tell if someone else is joking, will believe pretty much anything I am told, and yet refuse to believe that something has been said as a joke when I'm told that it is.

Something that often comes up in my conversations with autistic women about the causes of their frustrations is why people say they will do something and then don't do it or do something else. This is described as being 'literal' and seen as problematic, but the confusing part is that in the neurotypical world, the norm is to not expect things to be as they have been stated to be, which is entirely bizarre as a given. The discrepancy between people's words and actions is not only stressful due to the change in expectations that has to be processed (hard work), but also because it is not true and therefore illogical. There is nothing that stresses an autistic person more than a lack of logic or an unnecessary lie – we find it baffling. The unanswerable question of autism, which is always accompanied by a creased forehead, is: 'Why do people do that?' I once (jokingly) said at a conference that I wanted the forehead crease so often seen in autistic women to be called 'Hendrickx syndrome'. This talk was filmed and put onto YouTube. Since then, so many women have contacted me to tell me that this is also true of them, that perhaps I should pursue this route to infamy. My partner is constantly smoothing out the crease on my forehead. He says I have two facial expressions: puzzled and surprised.

Having their own words and motivations so frequently misunderstood leads autistic women to self-censorship, requiring them to be on 'red alert' to every single thought before they utter it. Even with this filter in place, social *faux pas* are common because the filter itself does not know what to look for. This fear is not social anxiety disorder in the sense that it is irrational and psychological in origin. The fear is based on evidence and fact and is wholly rational: it happens frequently and is due to a lack of typically expected cognitive skills in this area.

Managing uncertainty

Surprisingly, given the often independent and apparently functioning lives (as parents, academics and employees) that the women participants lead, their struggles with changes of plans and breaks to routines are significant. You would often never know that these women are finding things so tough. Their tendency is to tell the world that this new situation is fine, take the stress on themselves and do what is required, but then go home and cry and/or engage in self-destructive behaviours. I hate it when people change plans, but I never let it show because I'm supposed to be flexible. This leads people to think that I can handle anything. I tell them it's fine, but it's not fine. It's never fine. When they have gone my head hurts with the effort of making sense of why they couldn't do what they said they were going to do, what it will mean for me to have to reconfigure everything to take into account the new situation, and what bad things I can wish upon them for being so unreliable.

Mental and physical health conditions are the outcome of this refusal to admit limitations and maintain the façade of capability. Pushing oneself beyond what is comfortable to the point of illness can be an everyday occurrence, in order to avoid the admission of limitations that equates to failure for many autistic women. Admitting vulnerability and asking for concessions or help is hard after a lifetime of masking, especially when, before the realization of being autistic/diagnosis, you didn't know what it was that you needed help with or why: 'Other people can manage to lead a "normal" life, so why can't I?' The general assumption that most women I speak to have is that they were the problem and that they just needed to try harder.

> Dislike of changes to plans or vague plans when trying to plan outfit/shoes/things appropriate to activity/location/weather – intense dislike of feeling wrongly dressed or not having the right things with me.

> Changes, even minor ones, to routines upset me greatly and cause my behaviour to become challenging [...] A few weeks ago I had a meltdown because my mum was home half an hour late from walking the dog and I had planned to do something at

> that time, and losing that half-hour threw me out of my routine and ruined my whole day. She bore the brunt of my anger; it's a good thing she loves me unconditionally.

> I came home to find we had a new sofa, and the old one was outside in the yard. Again I went mad and went and sat on the old one in the yard, claiming I was going to live outside. Again I didn't understand my reaction, but it was very strong and I was horrible to my mum about it.

> I don't do change at all! It's just no. It doesn't work, it's like it should be A, B, C, D. If you go from A to D and miss out B and C, my brain shuts down. (Kock, Strydom, O'Brady and Tantum, 2019, p.15 [downloaded version])

> I need time to transition between places. Whenever I drive to a place where I'll need to be social, I spend a few minutes alone in my parked car before I go on. I spend this time shifting my expectations from the safety of solitude to the possibility of surprises. (Kotowicz, 2022, p.29)

> If I have leftover rice and I decide dinner tomorrow is fried rice, I react badly if someone eats my cooked rice, because I know the difference between fresh rice and leftover rice, and I wanted the leftover rice fried. I have also gone to bed hungry because of this. If I even try to avoid getting upset and 'just make something else', the frustration from cooking or thinking about another meal will cause a panic attack, and I won't be able to eat it after I'm done cooking it.

Like the autistic girls, the women maintain routines and schedules that ensure a level of certainty and predictability in their lives. These things provide structure and limit stress and anxiety. They should not be seen as a problem unless they are so restrictive that they are detrimental to a woman living her life and her ability to function. Many women adhere to a number of routines and procedures throughout their day, but these will not be immediately obvious and may be deliberately hidden. I will not answer the door or the phone if I don't know who it is. I am seen as a very able and independent person, but I suffer extreme anxiety at the prospect of leaving the house, even to go to the local shop. I have developed strategies to hide this from other people. It is surprisingly easy to maintain a required structure without anyone being aware that I am enabling my own need for predictable outcomes. The majority of NT individuals are not terribly observant when it comes to recognizing that someone in the office always wears the same clothes every Tuesday or drinks their tea from a specific mug. Maintaining these small measures may make the difference between an autistic woman feeling secure and able to cope with her day or feeling completely overwhelmed and ineffective because her markers of certainty have been lost. Some found relatively ordinary everyday expectations impossible to deal with and were inventive in finding their own solutions to these problems, often silently and alone without support.

> My whole life revolves around routines [...] I go through phases of obsessiveness, so I might eat the same food over and over again for weeks and then change. I get stuck on a song and replay it over and over again. These issues have always been the same throughout my life. I don't see it as a problem.

> Getting dressed and washed is difficult for me. I get things in the wrong order or might miss something out altogether, like forgetting to wash my armpits or something. To deal with this I have very strict routines: I wash my body in exactly the same way every time [...] If I get interrupted though, it's a different matter [...] If I reached for the shampoo and the bottle wasn't where it should be, I would find it very difficult to deal with that.

> I see the world as a puzzle to be solved, and meticulous planning means I function well, though with more stress.

> I manage by means of a complex schedule and a series of lists. My short-term memory is terrible, and without this, I would not be able to function.

Intense interests

> *Special interests make me feel alive, like I'm connected to something bigger than I am. It feels like a totally immersive flow state where there are no other thoughts; it's like you're swimming in the interest and can't shift your focus off it. I have always felt very ashamed of my 'crazy/obsessive' nature but am learning to accept it's part of who I am and actually has served me very well indeed (not a quitter!).*
>
> Steph Jones, autistic therapist and author of *The Autistic Survival Guide to Therapy* (forthcoming)

As life gets in the way of the all-encompassing pursuit of passions and intense interests, these get side-lined by the need for domestic and occupational obligations, but they still exist. (Musicians/bands, TV shows, science fiction and video-gaming were all favourite interests among the women I questioned.) Reading and gathering knowledge about special interests (often carried over from childhood) was still a huge draw for these women. The intensity of interest is still as great as it is for males, but the form of the interest can differ. Rather than simply focusing on the story being told, it is the people in TV shows and movies that can become obsessions, as both the character and the actor themselves. However, the topics of the shows are often science fiction – in line with typical male interests. Many interests enjoyed by autistic women can appear as fairly common – soap operas, cooking, travel – but, again, the depth of knowledge and the diligence put into the learning is way in excess of a 'hobby'. Other topics which can become intense in the depth to which they are explored are practical: learning a language for a forthcoming holiday, researching specifications for any number of technical items including cars, headphones and washing machines, or becoming an expert in dog care for the arrival of a new puppy. Autistic women generally don't dabble: they dive, and they dive deeply and with great passion and joy at what their discoveries reveal.

> I have got into debt before in pursuit of my collecting. I set myself a weekly Amazon budget now (I will do without clothes/toiletries to buy my books) for my books to control this. The book thing has always been a special interest of mine [...] It's not just about the content of the book for me; I actually like the book itself. I only like paperbacks because I like to feel the smooth, cool embossed covers and I like to flick the pages. I like the way a book smells and looks when [it is] on a bookshelf.

> [...] World War I and World War II. I'm absolutely fascinated by them. My grandad on my mum's side was in the army. My other grandad...was a pilot and mechanic... I go around military places and collect bits like gas masks, bombs, shrapnel, etc.

> [...] Morbid curiosity about all things relating to death. Learned about death; different cultures' ideas of afterlife; medical explanations about cardiac arrest and brain death and the sequence of organs shutting down after death; neurological research about death and the loss of consciousness; any scientific basis for the idea of a soul or spirit or self beyond neurones. My most recent school project was a festival about death and funeral rites, learning different ways to die, the process of drowning to death vs bleeding to death vs dying in a fire vs asphyxiation... I've also been suicidal since young, so I think my fascination with death and what it means to die stemmed from my desire to end my own life but be super-well-informed in what that entails.

> BOYS! Limerence [an all-consuming infatuation for another person] for me has been part of my life since I was five years old, and spent 14 years crushing on a boy in my class. It happens all the time, but since my diagnosis I now no longer look

> at myself as some weird stalker weirdo, just someone who gets hyper-fixated.

Many women have said that their enthusiasm for the subject ends when they lose interest, and describe this as being sudden and without explanation, but my extensive exploration into this by asking numerous women about the nature of their passions suggests otherwise. My impression is that each interest has an end goal for the person which is usually functional or target-driven in nature. For example, I met a woman who started running. She became completely fixated on running, equipment, timekeeping and so on, and built up her fitness to the point that she ran a marathon, after which she never ran again because for her there was nothing left to achieve. Others go on to triathlons or ultra-marathons, or become fitness coaches; the goal is always personal. For others, interests are functional: I taught myself to crochet one type of stitch via YouTube because I wanted to make a blanket. During every waking hour over several months, I obsessively made a series of large, striped, coloured blankets using my one stitch, sometimes for eight hours at a time. I stopped crocheting because it made no logical sense to make more blankets than I could not gift, sell or use. Other women I have known have stopped their interest for similar reasons: because they knew all there was to know, because they no longer had the space for the materials or finished products, or because they had been to Italy/bought a cooker/fixed the leak and so didn't need to learn Italian/about cookers/plumbing any more.

The autistic mind is curious and wants to learn, gather new knowledge and make connections between pieces of information. The new interest offers a steep and exciting trajectory of knowledge, which sadly at some point plateaus when competence, completion or success is achieved, or space and money have been depleted. To maintain the interest, what can work for some people is to take it sideways. For example, one young woman was deeply interested in Sherlock Holmes, which started with one TV series starring Benedict Cumberbatch, moving on to an earlier movie series starring Robert Downey Jr, then to the original Conan Doyle books and to individual actors, which linked her on to other projects that they had undertaken. Benedict Cumberbatch also played Dr Strangelove in the Marvel Universe, which led her deep into this series of movies, comic books and characters. Crafting interests can follow a similar sideways path: one woman started by taking up knitting. Once she had mastered every stitch, this led her to design her own patterns and spinning her own wool, eventually making a career as a knitting pattern designer. Perhaps before giving up on an interest that no longer excites and stimulates, it may be possible to consider what else could be done with these skills or materials. Or just move on to the next one with not a shred of guilt if you prefer.

What comes across in the women's words is often a sense of acceptance of their 'obsessions' that has accompanied their diagnosis of autism. Where previously they were embarrassed by the depth of their enthusiasms or their rapidly changing nature, the understanding of this type of behaviour being entirely typical within an autistic context appears to allow an enjoyment of the interests within the guilt and shame that may have previously tainted the joy.

My interests tend to be very, very short-lived. I will research for hours and hours and then get bored, sometimes even in the same day. I get an idea in my head and think it's the best thing ever, talk at length about it and then a week later forget it was even a thing! I have started degrees that I have never finished, and bought expensive fitness clothing or crafting things that I have never used... It almost feels like the idea of something and the research of it are more important and interesting than actually doing the activity. I also want to be the best at everything, and when I realize that this takes time and effort, I switch off from it. I doubt I will ever change, and I am at peace with that now.

> [...] This is really hard because I have *had* and *have* so many [interests]. I don't know how to do this. Is it dinosaurs? *Yes*. Is it anthropology? *Yes*. Is it singing? *Yes*. Is it colouring? *Yes*. Did I have all the crayons as a child? *Yes*. Do I have all the crayons *now*? *Yes*. They are just more expensive. Do I talk about

> everything all the time? Is it annoying to others? *Yes*. What is the trigger? Don't know. What are the emotions? Joy. Happiness. Is it negative? Maybe. But who cares...

Sensory experience

> I have this one favourite tree, and I'm going to sit under it for a few hours... I think this would help us all. To remember that it doesn't always have to feel bad to hear everything and see everything and smell everything. (Neville, 2019, p.31)

The sensory tolerance differences in autistic individuals are well reported and combine the experiences of feeling a strong need to either seek or avoid different sensory stimuli. The most commonly mentioned issues were crowded places and situations that were overwhelming from a holistic sensory perspective, rather than because of one particular sensory stressor.

> I hardly ever feel completely at ease in my body. Usually, something is too cold or too hot, too wobbly or too firm, too tight or too loose: it's very rare for everything to feel just right. (Kotowicz, 2022, p.20)

> I aim to be comfortable at all times: I can't stand to be in tight clothing, brightly lit rooms; even a crumb in the bed will kill me. I can no longer go to the supermarket because it's too overwhelming, and things must be 'just right' otherwise they are completely *wrong*.

> I pick up every stimulus in my brain. Everything is equal priority. A normal person's brain takes a frequency-locked loop of priority. (*Author's note: Google this phrase for clarity*)

Heightened sensory responses were not always perceived as negative – many autistic women report a wonderful intensity of sensation and attention to stimuli that those without autism do not have, and this brings them huge pleasure. Feeling particularly in tune with visual beauty and nature was a common theme.

> I have major problems with light [...] I do not like unexpected touch and will flinch, push away or go rigid when others touch me [...] Smells make me retch, quiet noises like leaves rustling or birds tweeting engulf my brain. However, I do feel blessed because although the unpleasant stuff is heightened, so is the good stuff. Certain music makes my brain dance [...] I feel very attached and deeply moved by the beauty of nature too.

> I wouldn't change it for the world really. It's just like vibing in a whole different place than other people and I can't help thinking I've got more in common with my cat's view of experiencing the world than the average Joe. I think it unlocks us to a magical world most people miss.

> I feel (music) more intensely than other people I think: to put headphones in is almost more euphoric than a lot of people would experience. (Milner *et al.*, 2019, p.2397)

Despite these positive sensory perceptions that bring great peace and joy, it is rare to find an autistic woman who doesn't require adjustments to her environment in one or more ways. Often these adjustments have been in place for many years prior to any inkling about autism being the root cause. Individuals have seen themselves as highly sensitive and been aware of these differences but not known why.

Noise

> Noise-cancelling headphones have changed my life when outside the home. I feel like I am I a cocoon when wearing them... I have been known to wear them in the cinema to lessen the noise levels.

Light/visual

> I used to think I had some kind of gifted eyesight, noticing things that other people can't see. I now realize that I'm just a garden variety autistic. I carried out an experiment with my ex-partner to describe what he saw looking at a plan door (I saw every detail like a bullfrog on acid). He saw a door.

> I have been diagnosed with Meares–Irlen syndrome and should wear blue-tinted glasses. I find screens difficult to look at, and they give me awful eye strain and headaches. When out of the house I will wear sunglasses even when it's cloudy, overcast or raining. On days where I am feeling especially tired/worn out, I will also wear them in shops or at home.

Touch

Touch - fabrics, people, surfaces - elicited the most responses as being a constant sensory challenge. From school uniforms to random hugs, the contact that one's body makes with the world is a significant source of distress and surveillance.

> I have a hard time with underwear because the tags and seams bother me so much all day until I rip them off, turn them inside out, or cry and take them off. I often wear my underwear inside out (and clothes too when I'm at home).

> I am highly reactive to most fabrics; I have cried from being forced to wear lace at family functions or to church with my family; I have taken off my clothes in restrooms of public spaces especially if I was having a panic attack. I have cried from laying on polyester satin bed sheets in hot, humid weather. I simply will not sleep on unevenly textured mattresses or sheets, pilling sheets, fabrics that retain moisture from sweat, etc... If I can't lay on a comfortable or even bearable surface to sleep, I will have suicidal thoughts all night.

> I can't sit on grass. Not in PE, not at a picnic, not at a park or at a party or in a sports tournament, not wild grass or freshly cut, watered grass, not with a thin picnic cloth/blanket and not even if the only alternative is to stand or squat all day. I just can't do it.

> A soft, light touch is incredibly painful to me, and a loose hair down my top can feel horrendous. Even the tiniest fleck of grit on my scalp feels like there's a million ants crawling in it, and people are often amazed when I find the offending microscopic particle and show them the damage it was causing.

> Before I found out that I take in more sensory data than most people, I wasn't able to explain how water affects me. My inner narrative didn't include the observation that rain hurts my skin, because every time I flinched at it, people would say, 'It won't hurt you'. (Kotowicz, 2022, p.21)

> Please don't touch me if you don't know me. Period.

> When clothes shopping, I will rub fabrics on my face and neck to see if they are scratchy or tickly.

> I am extremely ticklish, and if someone tickles me it can make me panic and cry. Therefore, I prefer firm touch and do find a tight hug from my partner incredibly relaxing.

> Whenever I worry that I am being ridiculous, my boyfriend Jake has a talent for helping me identify the valid logic that subconsciously drives my actions. Like, I felt silly packing twelve pairs of socks for a three-day trip, though he didn't see any problem with it. He reminded me that there's no sock police, but I needed to understand my motivation before I could accept it... We uncovered that my motivation was sensory – I didn't know which length and weight of socks the weather would require each day, and the wrong kind would have made me

> uncomfortable. To prevent that, I needed four pairs per day. (Kotowicz, 2022, p.25)

> Even thinking about touching velvet now makes me want to throw up.

Scratching, picking, rubbing, rocking, spinning and plucking hairs all featured as typical sensory behaviours. Many of these are not regarded as particularly unusual *per se*, but it is their intensity and frequency that demonstrate a difference. It is also the case that this type of behaviour is often attributed to anxiety disorders, but while this may be the case for autistic women, it also may not be. Autistic individuals are known to find solace and relaxation in repetitive movements, and therefore it should not automatically be assumed that behaviours of this type are a problem or only arise during anxiety. I find that picking and hair-pulling put me into a trance-like, almost meditative state, which is deeply relaxing and all-consuming. Understanding the function of the behaviour to the individual is necessary before suggesting it stops. Cessation without meeting that core need in some other less harmful way may provoke the inception of a new and more harmful physical response.

> I really, really enjoy spinning. I have a special spinny chair so that I can spin at home.

> [...] Tap foot or pat knee, press foot down to ground, flex arm tense so much to cause bruise on arm, squeeze jaw with cheeks pressed in, clench teeth, hold steering wheel very firmly.

> At times of stress I've found that plucking hairs out of my legs is very therapeutic. I don't think this is really self-harming; it only hurts a bit.

> I leave scratch marks all over my body, especially my chest, upper abdomen and lower back because I start massaging my skin every time I take off my clothes (the fabric is uncomfortable);

> and a massage turns into a high-pressure rub, and I activate my skin into feeling itchy which turns into light scratching, which then turns into vigorously scratching my skin. By the following day, my skin is sore, there are scratch marks and scabs all over me, and pouring water on my skin hurts.

Smell

As with other sensory stimuli, smells are either sought or avoided with some describing a great sense of calm when smelling a beloved scent, whether it be flowers or bleach. Others found everyday smells, perfumes and products unbearable to the point of being unable to function in their presence and/or needing to leave the location.

> If I had lilies in the house, she'd go almost deaf...it was like the sensory overload made something else shut down. (Milner *et al.*, 2019, p.2397)

> I hate aerosol deodorants, body sprays and air fresheners...and make quite a fuss about having to open windows.

> I carry a bottle of lavender essential oil spray everywhere I go. Whenever I am overwhelmed by smells around me – which I seem to notice far more than other people – I mask them with my spray and then I can cope.

Temperature

> Hot temperature makes me so angry I can get aggressive. I once came out of the gym (too hot) and started kicking a wheelie bin.

> I can't cope with the cold. This makes me shiver extremely badly. If I go out, I have six pairs of socks on, two T-shirts and two jumpers and a thick coat on top.

> I have hurt myself by accident many times by showering with hot

> water over 50 degrees Celsius or cold water under 10 degrees, regardless of the weather. I lived in an apartment that showed the water temperature, and there were days when anything less than 50 was not hot enough and anything above 10 was not cold enough.

Sharing

As discussed in Chapter 3, in childhood autistic females have difficulties with the concept of sharing, and for some that doesn't go away. They may have learned that sharing is something that is required and will concede without complaint, but that does not mean that it comes easily. Lending or sharing an item means a loss of control and not knowing where that item is (as well as knowing that it is not where it is supposed to be), along with a feeling of insecurity and potentially an additional social interaction that has to be managed delicately (mental effort): 'How will I get it back?' This is associated with a preference for routine, sameness and a dislike of change – specifically, change that is imposed by others. All of these elements encompass the same basic stressors: 'I don't know how to make sense of this and how to maintain control'. Controlling possessions, tasks and environments reduces stress and anxiety. Autistic women are generally not team players and prefer to go it alone when doing tasks and projects since other people involve sharing ideas, and hence compromise and more communication to reach a consensus, when she could have just done it all herself.

The sharing of space when co-habiting causes issues. For me one of the key factors in my own ability to function well is knowing where every single item I possess is – always. I never need to worry about not having what I need or having to look for it. I know where to find what I will require at any given moment in time; therefore, stress regarding this matter is reduced to zero. Living with other people means that things are moved. The impact of this is huge for me – far greater than simply the annoyance of having to look for or ask for something. The certainty of my personal physical world is the foundation of my existence, and it is hard for others to understand that my extreme distress and blinding headache at someone having moved the sticky tape is not an over-reaction or a sign of mental illness: it's all an easily explainable part of being autistic.

> [...] Very wary of lending people anything, even in the event of loaning something as meagre or trivial as a pencil. Far too aware of the time that each person spent with a loaned item as well, and would be combative if someone was notably 'hogging' something for long periods when compared with the rest of those concerned.

> I do not share. Over the years, for the few times I have shared, I have learned that I will never get whatever I shared back in any form, nor will the kindness be reciprocated at any point in time.

> I hate people to be in my space and my stuff [...] When I moved in with my husband, I completely freaked out for at least a year. He is now well and truly part of the furniture!

> I don't like sharing my stuff. I don't like sharing my space. I am willing to do it for someone I like but it doesn't feel less troubling. I just choose to accept the disturbance for certain people, but when I share my things or space with someone I like and it is clear that it is in fact a disturbance, people get offended or feel hurt because they believe like it shouldn't *feel* the same for a stranger, but it does. I simply choose who is worth the disturbance and hope they don't move a single inch beyond what I consented to, which causes problems too because people feel too comfortable around friends and family.

Fantasy worlds

The fantasy world described in the childhood experiences of autistic girls still exists for a number of adult women, and why wouldn't it? The escape from a difficult world that imaginary worlds offered her childhood self is needed just as much in adult life. The processing and running-through of events and scenarios may be a useful strategy for making sense of situations, and providing respite from a life that does not offer the emotional highs and predictability of the literature that many of these girls and women have been reading voraciously since childhood. Real life is dull and scary by comparison. Unless there is a genuine concern that the person cannot determine fantasy from reality and is in danger of harm, I would argue that these worlds and characters play a valuable role for autistic women in coping with life and should be accepted for what they are.

> I currently only have one imaginary friend, who takes the form of my late best friend/love. He often works as my common sense when I'm deep in anxiety, reassuring me that the things I think are just warped perceptions. I will often talk to him out loud.

> [...] Fantasize about living in a different part of the country and starting over, kind of like witness protection, cutting all ties to my present life [...] like a new identity.

> I assumed the persona of many an alternate being when feeling overwhelmed or threatened. My perception of my surroundings would be engulfed by the sensations I imagined my 'other me' would experience. It was essentially an alternate universe. This fantasy world persists to this day, and my need to re-imagine the mundane.

> I never had imaginary friends, but [from] a teenager onwards I did have imaginary lovers. I dreamed up plenty [of] imaginary worlds. I love fantasy literature and that has continued to fuel those imaginary worlds.

Clothes

Something I noted in the autistic girls was their choice of clothing, which was selected for function rather than fashion. For many of the women questioned, this remains the case. Unless fashion is a specific interest or passion, it is largely irrelevant to the majority of autistic women I have met. Some women described an androgynous appearance and choice of clothing; others had strong preferences for certain colours, textures or styles. Plain, in general, was preferred to anything overly ornate or fussy; and if something fits and works, buying a number of the same item (possibly in different colours if she is feeling particularly frivolous) makes logical sense. Shoes, handbags, jewellery and other accessories are not something that I see on most of the autistic women that I meet.

> My clothes are very samey and simple [...] My husband thinks I am hilarious and brilliant at the same time. I am in and out of the shops in a flash. My new winter coat this year was virtually identical to last year's; he laughed so much when he saw it.

> I tend to wear simple clothing that could just as easily be worn by a man (albeit a small one). Of course I am aware of gender expectations and will wear high heels if the occasion requires it, although I think that even when I dress feminine, my style is always a little bit manly.

> If I find something I like that fits and that doesn't hurt, I will buy several. I feel a palpable sense of relief when this happens, knowing that I don't have to go through the whole process again anytime soon because I am now sorted for some time.

Chapter 5

LATER YEARS

> *Having a late diagnosis helps enormously with coming to terms with my past, adapting how I live now, and hopefully guiding decisions about the future.*
>
> Autistic woman, diagnosed aged 68 years

The first generation of children diagnosed as autistic in childhood during the 1940s are only now approaching their elder years, and in light of this the National Autistic Society has developed the Autism in Maturity project to address the issues that these individuals may face. It is not only those diagnosed in childhood who make up this ageing autistic population: 71 per cent of autistic individuals over the age of 55 received their diagnosis in the past decade (National Autistic Society, 2013b).

In general, autism research has excluded individuals over 40 years of age, and little is known about what will happen to older adults as they age, with even less known about women specifically. Michael (2015) contacted people in the autism research community asking for news of any known or future studies focusing on older autistic women and found none – either past, present or planned. Beyond 40 years of age, it would appear that we don't exist. There has been some progress since then, but not a great deal. There is some interesting work being carried out into autistic menopause (discussed later in this book) – and a small number of studies have been undertaken to look at social cognitive abilities in all genders of autistic people, and some have found that the decline is slower than in the neurotypical population, such as category learning and numerical pattern completion (Charlton, 2017) – but there are no long-term longitudinal studies examining the neurocognitive profile of ageing in autistic people (Happé and Charlton, 2012). One study looked at 15 cognitive outcome measures over a 3.5-year period with participants ranging from 24 to 85 years of age (Torenvliet *et al.*, 2023). They found that there were no significant differences between the autistic and non-autistic participants, which is encouraging, but in short, it is fair to say that we simply don't yet know what will happen to us.

> I have read books by other Aspies and trawled the Internet forums. There is a lot of emphasis on young autistic people. I was never a young person with autism, as I had no idea I had it. I was a young person with problems. I am now a middle-aged woman learning for the first time to recognise my problems as Aspie problems and look for interventions. I have the problems, but there don't seem to be any interventions available to people of my age. (National Autistic Society, 2013a)

Given that around the majority of the participants in the research for this book were in their 40s and above – and most of those were only diagnosed in the last few years – we have a population of women moving towards their elder years, the majority of whom have only just discovered who they are.

> I did not know that I was autistic as a child, young person, teenager, young adult or middle-aged person. That has been all a process of retrospect, of looking backwards in dozen upon dozen 'aha' moments. Some are kind of numbing to think about. Life might have been easier with some kind of intervention on my Aspie behalf.

We know that in general terms we are an ageing population and that support and services for growing numbers of older people will be increasingly necessary in years to come. What we don't really know is what impact ageing has on autistic people. What we do know is that only a small number of autistic adults are 'ageing well'. The definition of ageing well has been a popular concept since the 1980s and includes the criteria of avoiding disease and disability, and maintaining high physical and cognitive functioning and active engagement with life. When applying these criteria to autistic adults, researchers found that only 3 per cent were ageing well. They propose that the standard criteria for ageing well may not be entirely applicable to autistic older people and that a more inclusive and autism-specific model may be required, which is not so deficit-based or subjective by neurotypical givens of what quality of life looks like (Hwang, Foley and Trollor, 2020).

> Life with autism is more difficult as I get older. I realize that life as anyone gets older is more difficult. Instead of just letting it happen and be poorly adjusted to, why not strive to make it the best transition it can be? A positive outlook and some good choices can make the difference. Decide to be a role model to younger people and autistic people. They need to know that getting older can be a good thing.

Suggested priorities for autistic women include research on support for bereavement, independent living and the effects of menopause (Michael, 2015).

These insights are important because, in stating the obvious, every autistic girl will eventually become an autistic older woman, and if we know what to watch out for, we can start the process early to minimize the negative effects.

The positive aspects of growing older

I got a real sense that the older autistic women had been able to come to terms with who they are. Due to their often very late diagnosis, self-acceptance had not been possible earlier in their lives. They talked about being able to assert what they needed to maintain their own well-being, and feeling okay about that, rather than feeling bad about being perceived as different or difficult, which had been the case pre-diagnosis. After a lifetime of not being listened to, taken seriously or believed, some women were also able to obtain correct medication for their anxiety, depression and/or associated health conditions, which made life much easier. Having time to look after their health and well-being was also mentioned as being a positive result of becoming older.

> I am still very much a creature of habit and love routine. My ability to deal with change has improved a great deal as I have a better sense of perspective about what is the 'small stuff' that doesn't really matter.

> I allow myself to be more and more myself in public and ask for things that suit me. If that means that I'm going to be that eccentric, odd old lady, who no one understands, so be it!

> I find it's more important than ever to have my home as a place of sanctuary. I need to have things around me which make me feel calm and happy [...] I think this is especially important the older you get. When the door buzzer goes, I ignore it when I want. The same goes for my telephone. If I don't feel like answering, I leave it. Email suits me just fine as it's not an intrusion into my peace and I can reply when I feel like it. (National Autistic Society, 2013a)

> My health has improved as I've got older, partly due to correct medication and more recently due to taking up a fairly intensive gym regime. I'm fitter than I've ever been and hope to maintain that as the years go by.

> I'm finding that being an older woman in today's society renders me somewhat invisible, especially as I don't conform to my gender stereotype by wearing overtly feminine clothes and make-up, and I find this invisibility a relief and advantageous in that I have less unwelcome, intrusive attention to deal with.

For some older autistic women there is a sense of feeling comfortable with themselves for the first time (Simone, 2010) and feeling more able to be their 'real' selves, almost becoming 'more autistic' in the process. Several women mentioned that they felt this way and that this had been surprising both to their families and the professionals around them. They felt that others had expected them to become more 'normal' and that this had not happened (Simone, 2010). This was combined with the physical and mental decline in function mentioned above: 'I can't do it any more; I don't want to do it any more'. Eccentricities became more pronounced, and tolerances were reduced. Some mentioned feeling younger than their age and, perhaps due to a lesser need to conform to social norms, being able to engage in activities and with people not traditionally associated with older women. Autistic women often don't see any reason why they shouldn't do something due to age, gender or any other factor. This is enormously liberating and the reason why you'll find older autistic women doing all sorts of crazy stuff!

> I now go to roller discos and find it has really cheered me up as most of the people there are a bit younger than me. There are some people older too though, so I'm not like the odd one out or anything. It's good to keep joining things that are not just for older people.

> I still feel and act much younger than my age. If I am talking to women in their 20s I feel I can laugh at silly things, and if I can have a bit of a lark playing a game of ten-pin bowling with a group of 25-year-old Aspie girls then I feel so much better afterwards. (National Autistic Society, 2013a)

> God, what a relief being older is. I've become invisible. No one expects anything of me any more – I'm just old. Sad though that is in some ways, it's also a huge liberation: I can do whatever I like, and nobody cares.

> There are problems I haven't been able to rectify, but I know how

> to be kind to myself. When I get home, electric lights go off and I light candles. I burn oils because they calm me. I am learning how to slow down the chatter that runs through my head and I am looking for the key to a full night of sleep. I might never be at ease with you, but I am more at ease with myself. (National Autistic Society, 2013a)

Susan Moreno, in her article 'Autism After 65: Making the Most of the Golden Years' (Moreno, 2018) suggests ways of supporting older autistic people. She advocates the need to appreciate the gifts and skills of the person, and that engaging their interests and knowledge is a way to make a person feel more valuable. Susan also notes that autistic people may find it difficult to communicate their specific concerns or changes. For example, rather than noting they cannot see or hear as well as they used to, they may comment that someone changed the light bulbs for dimmer ones or turned the volume of the TV down, when neither thing has occurred. Susan also reminds those supporting older autistic people of the 'not about me, without me' ethos and ensuring that the person's idea of quality of life, preferred routines and sensory needs are paramount in their care, especially at the point in their lives when they may be reliant on others to advocate for these on their behalf.

Physical and mental effects of autistic ageing

Common features mentioned by older women were tiredness and fatigue. Although this is something generally associated with ageing, it appears that this perhaps comes on slightly earlier for autistic women – by the age of 40 – despite them being in otherwise good physical health. For some, getting through a whole day was too much without a nap. I am 100 per cent with them on this point and find the physical limitations that have come on quite quickly with ageing are both frustrating and a glorious liberation.

> I have needed a sleep in the afternoon since being around age 40.

> My health is good and I'm very fit for my age, but I get so tired and often have to fall asleep for a few hours in the daytime.

> I'm forcing myself to exercise regularly and stretch my mental limits by studying a new language to ward off needing physical or mental care.

Along with a general physical tiredness, a number of women I have worked with have expressed a tiredness of holding it all together, of pretending to be someone else, of masking their autism. There is a real sense that the effort that these women have been making since childhood may have some long-term toll. They run out of steam; they simple can't do it any more (or don't want to). The words used talk of fighting to 'survive': these women have been battling to keep going in a world that feels alien and difficult. It seems that the combination of physical limitations associated with ageing and the number of years they have been 'fighting' can lead to a gradual slow-down once they reach their 40s and beyond.

> I was getting older, and instead of things getting easier for me they were becoming more difficult as I had additional health issues to deal [with] (asthma, migraine disorder, hypothyroidism, IBS [irritable bowel syndrome], neuropathy, etc.). This constant stress was causing other health issues, including depression, and an overall lack of desire to live. I was just getting extremely tired of it all and tired of the fight to survive. My life was just one crisis after another.

> I am tired of playing the role of someone who fits in, someone who can hold down a job and who wants what everyone else wants. I never wanted any of those things; I just did what I had to do to survive unnoticed and uncriticized. It has destroyed me mentally – and physically to some extent. I just want to retreat and live a small, quiet life. I've had enough.

> Lack of energy as I get older has limited the interests I pursue;

> this is disappointing, as there are many things that I have really enjoyed doing. Part of this, of course, is the depression that comes with Asperger's. Curtailing activities is par for the course. In an effort to get this energy back, I have started to exercise daily and work on my eating plan.

> Being in crowds stresses me, like in a town, although it never used to. I don't know if the crowds have got bigger or if the older I've got my brain's processing of their movements has slowed down. I seem to find I use up so much energy trying to move among people.

> I think I have gotten less interested in fitting in, less able to bite my tongue, less aware of gaffes, more tired, and far more resistant to change and unable to cope.

Other physical limitations mentioned mostly involved memory and a feeling of reduced brain-processing ability and speed.

> One of the less positive things about my age is that the rate at which my brain processes information seems to have slowed down. I feel as if I have constant 'brain fog'. It seems to take [...] much longer for my brain's processing ability to kick in when I wake up. (National Autistic Society, 2013a)

> I can't remember facts at all, or names or people, places, TV programmes, characters in them or anything, and have got worse since reaching middle age.

> [...] Use [my] index finger to point at objects or directions to help [my] brain know what to do. For instance, when at the grocery store I use my index finger to point at objects I'm trying to look for so I don't miss something I need to buy. When driving, I use my index finger to point at the direction I need to turn.

> When I'm busy doing some activity, like getting ingredients

> together for a recipe, I can't respond to someone's question or conversation. I have to concentrate on doing what I'm doing to get it right. The same is also true when I'm typing an email to someone dear. I can't respond to someone's question or conversation.

A couple of women mentioned having increasing difficulties with speech.

> I am finding it harder to speak coherently. Quite often I will say the wrong word or a made-up word, or I stutter. I have always been very strong linguistically, and I find this upsetting and frightening as I don't know how it will progress. I am only in my 40s. [...] At times I say partial sentences, like that's all I can get out. My husband understands me, but I wonder if others would. When around other people, I usually just don't say anything unless I can speak with whole sentences.

Other physical changes mentioned included eyesight and hearing problems (which may be a natural consequence of ageing). These may have an additional impact for an autistic person who does not recognize faces well and has to look for other visual cues, or for someone who has always struggled to filter noise in busy environments. The loss of these faculties can greatly increase anxiety and make a person reluctant to leave the house and maintain an active life.

> My eyesight causes me a lot of stress as I have so many pairs of glasses and forget them half the time [...] I mess about with a magnifying glass in the house to read labels on food as I can't locate my reading specs.

> Hearing in large crowds is always difficult. It is hard to focus on what the one person is saying when you really hear all the other voices at the same time. Sometimes I find myself cupping my hand over the back of my ear to hear better.

Accessing health and social care in later years

Autistic individuals are known to have differences in the way that they experience and report pain (National Autistic Society, 2013b). This may mean that they do not alert professionals when they are unwell. They also may have more limited family and social networks, which could mean that their poor health goes unnoticed for considerable periods of time. For non-verbal autistic people, this difficultly can exhibit as challenging behaviour and the underlying health problems go unaddressed. Care must be taken to ensure that older autistic people are sufficiently monitored, particularly if they live alone in the community.

> I don't experience pain in the same way as other people [...] I can open up the oven, pick up a cast-iron casserole, stand up with it, put it on the table, and it's only when my niece says, 'Auntie, your hands are peeling off,' that I think, 'This isn't good', but it'll be another five minutes before mild discomfort becomes agony. I missed appendicitis completely and woke up in hospital with peritonitis. (Nancy, in National Autistic Society, 2013a)

Accessing health care for individuals who experience anxiety and difficulties with new situations may be exacerbated in older life when accompanied by dementia, hearing loss, memory loss and poor eyesight. Training for healthcare professionals is essential in ensuring that distress is minimized for these individuals and that care is made accessible. It is also essential that domiciliary and residential home care workers understand the profile of the autistic person and do not inadvertently cause stress by not recognizing the person's needs.

> I think that having the diagnosis will help me understand that communal living isn't going to be my preferred option. I need my personal space and down time, so my current situation is perfect for that. If I need care at any point, I guess the best option will be carers visiting as necessary.

> I have Power of Attorney signed and sealed with my brother and nephews, and I shared my diagnosis with the family because it will possibly impact on decisions that they might have to make for me in the future.

> In all events, I will fight to stay in my own home. Having to live in a nursing facility, with a constant rotation of staff and pressure of shared experiences and dining, would be misery for me.

> The staff in the care home where my mum is staying don't stick to time, come into her room without asking, don't tell her if builders are coming in to change the carpets or move furniture, and don't do what they've said they will. She hates it. (Adult daughter of older autistic woman)

> As a society the very young and the very old get more than their fair share of physical contact, because neurotypicals want to pat them. I saw some excellent carers [...] who, when they spoke to someone who was a bit vague, the hand would go down and they'd say, 'How are you today Mrs Brown?' 'All right, yes', and they'd be hand-holding her. That's absolutely right for a neurotypical; it's absolutely wrong for an autistic person [...] The horror of unwanted physical contact with people [...] you know they're doing this to be nice, but their fingers feel like ice on me. That's horrible, and so stressful. Some of the most stressful and distressing things neurotypicals do is hug. (Lillian, in National Autistic Society, 2013a)

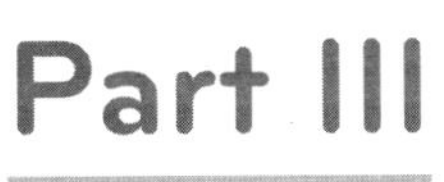

FACETS OF LIFE

Chapter 6

SOCIAL RELATIONSHIPS

It is a widely held view that autistic individuals have a different understanding and requirement for social interactions from neurotypical people, and being a 'loner' is often considered part of the autism profile. This is not always the case, and some autistic females are extremely proactive in seeking social connections, but these efforts are not always well received if directed towards a neurotypical audience that does not understand or appreciate their different communication style.

Childhood relationships

From the participants' responses, 50 per cent were considered 'shy' as young children, a view that is also found in the literature (Giarelli *et al.*, 2010; Riley-Hall, 2012). A small number fell into the 'overpowering' category, where the wants of the other children were not taken into consideration; but in general, these girls were quiet – unusually quiet. This quietness does not alert professionals to any potential difficulties: quiet is harmless and isn't causing any trouble.

> Being alone did not really bother me – I was happy with my own company. One thing that did disturb me was how other people seemed to enjoy each other's company and actively sought friendships and relationships. (Lawson, 2000, p.57)

> Both at school and at home I try to spend as much time alone

> as I can 'cause it...gets me in a very calm state of mind so that when I do need to interact with people I'm willing to talk and socialise and stuff. (Milner *et al.*, 2019, p. 2395)

One study (Head *et al.*, 2014) of 100 children using the Friendship Questionnaire (FQ) developed by Baron-Cohen and Wheelwright (2003), which measures friendship quality, understanding and empathy, found that autistic girls scored similarly to non-autistic boys and higher than autistic boys. This finding may support explanation of camouflaging in autistic females in that although the girls' social performance may be 'superficially level' to their non-autistic female peers, their actual understanding of friendships may be considerably lower.

For some autistic girls, their proactive sociability can be a clue to their neurodivergent nature in itself. It is possible to be *too* sociable (according to expected norms), with too few boundaries and little understanding of the feelings and intentions of neurotypical others. Females on the autism spectrum span the social range from those who don't want to engage at all or who actively avoid interaction, to those who have a strong desire for interaction but who don't know what to say and when to stop talking. The skills involving theory of mind and the development of intuitive empathy are not developed until around four years of age in typically developing children, and so cannot be indicative of potential autism in a child under this age.

> She is incredibly sociable and seeks interaction with anyone she meets [...] With adults it can make her vulnerable – she wanted to cuddle the telephone engineer and the dog food delivery man (when she was six or seven) [...] when she 'takes a shine' to someone, she will not be swayed. (Parent)

> When I did interact, it was inappropriate. For example, as a young toddler I would sometimes seek out physically stimulating activities or rough play with certain adults, such as rubbing up against them, rocking in their lap, seeking to have my back

> or my arms scratched or tickled, roughly playing with their hair or their hands, etc.

> Imagine an introverted machine. It charges by being on its own. And then me: an extrovert machine charged by being around people but with an introvert operating system. I hate meeting new people but feel energized by them when I do.

Difficulty understanding the rules and expectations of social situations is a common feature of autism, and one that requires not only verbal and non-verbal interpretation and expression, but also a kind of cultural understanding of what is required and expected in any given, specific setting. Autistic individuals may lack some of these subtle observational abilities and need more direct guidance in order to know how to act. It seems to me that autistic individuals have to learn mechanically (consciously) what others learn intuitively (unconsciously).

> I was constantly being trained by my mother on how to read the non-verbal cues of others and how to say the right things at the right time. We often role-played what to do and say in various situations. I was not very good at generalizing from one situation to the next. It's almost as if I had to know the specific script for each situation and encounter, no matter how similar the situations might be to a past experience.

> When my grandma died, everyone was crying, and I didn't understand why; I was seven or eight so I didn't really understand death, but I knew that she was 'gone' so I asked my sister why everyone is crying that she's 'gone', because she was mean, and we didn't like her. My sister responded that she was gone forever, and she would never come back. At which point (still not understanding why everyone is crying, *because she was mean and did not like us*), I asked for lunch and got told off. I still didn't understand the overt display of sadness or why I got told off for asking for food while people were crying (until I was older).

Again, for girls, the expectation is that they will be naturally good at this extremely subtle, intuitive, nuanced skill that requires adaption from moment to moment. For autistic females this cannot be assumed, and care should be taken not to reprimand an autistic girl more severely than one would an autistic boy behaving in a similar fashion. It is also important to recognize this behaviour in girls for what it is, rather than attribute it to another (perhaps intentional) reason. The girls in my survey describe friendships on their terms, sometimes with little perception or regard for the feelings of others, even after theory of mind had kicked in for their peers. These girls were making fewer – or at least more socially clumsy – attempts at connecting with peers from a very young age than would be expected from a typically developing child. Autistic girls are seen to have fewer and more intense friendships than their neurotypical peers, but more in line with their peers than with autistic boys (Sedgewick, 2018).

> A really wanted to relate to adults or older children. She didn't seem to 'get' how to be with her peers [...] She would rather hit someone over the head or cover them in paint, which didn't endear her to either them or their parents. (Parent)

> I certainly remember wondering, feeling like normal people have telepathy [*sic*], the ability to sort of telepathy, like telling each other in their minds what they had broadcast a telepathic message saying let's kick this friendship off by going to my house and having a party or something and...it's like I'm not telepathic: I can't pick up any telepathic messages. (Milner *et al.*, 2019, p.2398)

For most of the girls and women who participated in my research, there was some desire to interact with people, and often a sense of a conscious awareness of finding it difficult – despite the desire to do it – from a young age. They appeared to process the experience consciously rather than intuitively, observing the situation almost from a distance and working out what to do, but often missing some important element, for example what it is to have a friend and be a friend. This suggests that a huge amount of early awareness and cognitive processing are required. One can imagine that this would be isolating, exhausting and baffling for a young autistic child, and that they might also have a sense that everyone else just seems to 'get it'.

> Playtime was very difficult. I didn't know how other kids just sort of knew what to do and who to play with. So, I just hung out by myself, wandered around the playground, sometimes standing weirdly in a group of kids, not saying much, thinking that was enough to be included and considered a part of whatever game they were playing. Mostly I just watched.

> I remember feeling like I should play one-to-one, because no one else played alone, but I didn't know how to make it happen.

Certainly, some women were not forthcoming in seeking interaction and actively avoided doing so. Liane Holliday Willey (2014) recalls an overwhelming desire to be away from her peers in her earliest years, much preferring the company of her imaginary friends. In either case, whether silent or actively seeking an audience, most of the girls in my sample were typically not considered as potentially autistic until they had reached adulthood, despite what, with hindsight, can be seen as clear indicators of some difference. On reflection, it is easy to attribute their behaviour to shyness, or even high intelligence in some cases, but when combined with a broad profile and an understanding of autism, indications of their future diagnosis are not difficult to see.

> Other people are just walking noise machines. I didn't wish to be around them and desperately wanted to be alone much of the time.

> On my first day of kindergarten, I hid behind my mum's legs and stood with her and the other parents, staring at the kids. I had absolutely no desire to socialize with them or to play.

> Playtime for my daughter would consist of running up and down the perimeter of the fence, flapping and clapping her hands and having an inner dialogue with herself. (Parent)

Some of the women questioned had a strong sense of being tolerated by other children, rather than actively liked. The effect of this awareness must have had a considerable impact on self-esteem and well-being.

> I made a few friends from my class, all of whom bossed me around and eventually got sick of me. Whenever I didn't have any friends from my class, I'd play with kids from younger classes, but even they would eventually point out that I should play with kids my own age.

More than 25 per cent of the women questioned had experienced bullying as children. Bullying among the autistic population is old news, and it is rare in my work that I meet an autistic person who hasn't been bullied at school and beyond. It is possible that for some of these girls, their 'shyness', invisible presentation and quiet demeanour may have protected them from bullying to some degree. Perhaps those girls who were bullied were more obviously different in some way, which made them an easy target. Many of the responses give the impression that the girls were mostly simply left alone, as they were of very little interest to bullies (or anyone else for that matter), but, sadly, that wasn't always the case.

> I was constantly being bullied. A lot of the times even by the people I considered to be my best friends. I was picked last on the team, not invited to parties, called names, and once they even put glue on my chair.

> I did attach to the most 'high-status' group of friends at my primary school [...] as they served a purpose for me in reducing the bullying I faced [...] I wouldn't really call that 'friendship' though, it was more an interaction of convenience.

That is not to say that all autistic girls are the passive type. Some girls can be loud, outspoken and come across as aggressive or dictatorial, needing to control any interactions and struggling when games change or things don't go their way. The child can appear serious and intolerant of others whom they perceive are 'doing it wrong'.

> My sister says that when we were kids she was always under the impression that she was annoying me [...] I remember being very authoritarian and wanting to dictate to them [siblings] how to play.

For these girls their social difficulties can manifest in a more proactive, socially clumsy and sometimes overpowering way. Eileen Riley-Hall (2012) suggests that there is less tolerance from teachers for aggression in girls than in boys, and that girls, from an early age, are expected to be more polite and considerate of others' feelings.

> I was something of a tyrant [...] but only to those I viewed as wrongdoers. I had a keen sense of justice even at that age; but to those who ended up on my naughty list, so to speak, I would act almost animalistic towards them and was pulled out of the group for physical aggression.

> Sometimes I was a bully, especially when I spent time with younger kids. They would get me to go and hit a child they didn't like and this would make me popular with them, so I did it.

> I was quite violent, when I couldn't communicate what was wrong. I think I just let my fists do the talking.

Autistic girls may appear to have friends or, more accurately, often just one friend, so the child doesn't appear to be particularly isolated or a 'loner'. For some girls, this one friend can become a lifeline and help her to gain access into the social arena. The friend can become a subject of fascination and focus, which can cause enormous distress if and when she decides she wants to play with other children.

> From a very young age, I craved exclusivity with a 'best friend'.

> A lot of my problems came about with them having other friends that I didn't like or didn't get on with... I didn't really want to share them. (Bargiela *et al.*, 2016, p.3289)

In other cases, autistic women say that large groups were the best places for them, as they could hide on the peripheries with little requirement to participate (Attwood, 2007).

> Larger groups meant I could smile, laugh, agree and hide away, camouflaged by the group identity.

The girls' friends are sometimes very similar to them – other girls who find the social whirl difficult for various reasons – or they are very different: super-sociable girls who scoop up the stragglers and mother them. All of this leads the casual observer to conclude that all is well in the social world of the autistic girl.

> They [friends] were those that were considered outlandish for various reasons.

> I describe her [friend] as a 'social crutch'. (Parent)

> Her friends have been foreign children with a different language. (Parent)

The other common friends for autistic girls are boys. The vast majority of girls and autistic women that I spoke to identify themselves as 'tomboys' and/or find other girls to be far more complex and nuanced in their social skills than boys. This is particularly the case in the teenage years when friendships change from being interest-based to being more personality-based, and the autistic girl can struggle to keep up with the multiple and involved intricacies of female teenage relationships.

> I wanted to play with boys at school. I don't think I understood other girls and did not feel comfortable with them, always whispering and giggling. Girls are not nurturing; they are mostly bitchy and cliquey.

> I just feel so much more comfortable with men because they're more...you can take them at face value and it's not that fear of them judging you or having alternative motives and thoughts and they kind of say things straight. (Bargiela *et al.*, 2016, p.3289)

Seeking adult interaction, rather than peer interaction, from a young age appears to be a common feature of many girls on the autism spectrum, with around 60 per cent of those asked saying that adults were their first choice of companion. Mothers and grandparents were favourite companions, with some girls not requiring or seeking anyone in the world other than these people as a playmate.

> My daughter just wants to be with me. She tells me this all the time. (Parent)

> I rarely sought out people, and when I did it was for a specific task or to play a specific game or get help with a piece of work. I didn't ever seek out people just for idle chit-chat or to play their games or because I wanted a hug or any other such nonsense. I preferred the company of adults.

Adults feel less complicated than peers to engage with, and their communication is usually clearer. As a child, my preferred choice for my birthday party was an evening of card games with a family that my mum had known her entire life: two elderly parents and their adult children. I was the only child. I never had any birthday party other than this except to have a birthday tea with one other child – always the same food every year, which was of my choosing (ravioli, mash and peas followed by Swiss roll and evaporated milk). And I never wanted one. The idea of being the centre of attention in a social gathering of children would have been a horrific thought. The same applies to adult birthday parties now.

Masking and camouflaging in childhood

We have noted that autistic girls learn how to behave socially by observing and copying behaviour witnessed in others in order to appear socially typical. These girls may also practise these behaviours further through play with dolls and toys. When taking the role of a socially skilled girl, they may re-enact scenarios and conversations they have had or overheard. This role-play helps them to analyse and rehearse situations (Attwood *et al.*, 2006). The common interest of reading fiction seen in autistic girls is also a valuable tool in learning about communication and relationships. Later on in life, they may turn to psychology or self-help books for this data, but for now, Enid Blyton may well be the source of their social research.

> As a child, I kept a bank vault of phrases I heard from cartoons and shows that I liked or could relate to, and I used those phrases as responses in my conversation. I started adding song lyrics and lines from books and poetry into the vault in my pre-teens and early teens. This was used to express emotions if I felt I'd read or heard exactly what I wanted to say, said in a way that I couldn't have said or paraphrased better.

> She tried to make friends by watching and copying behaviour, but it never worked particularly successfully. (Parent)

> Mimicry is the word, although this was by no means a conscious effort. I even copy people's accents without myself knowing until the afterthought dawns on me in retrospect [...] I know I definitely was flagged a weirdo to the general populace. I guess I

> just didn't know. I can remember just sitting by a clique, which hopefully would not take offence to my mere presence, to pass by the more social times.

Adolescent relationships

> In the earlier years, I think I was too oblivious to social norms to notice how different I was or that I wasn't 'doing it right'. But the older I got, the more I started to feel different and anxious to be liked.

> I did not understand the girls' group dynamics. I was always on the periphery, and I felt very inadequate.

> I often felt as if I was peering in – looking at what others were doing, constantly observing actions and reactions. And so I learned to 'act normal'; and judging by people's reactions when I say I'm an Aspie, I'm a very good actress.

> I was unable to understand the inane 'rules' of teenage girls which meant I was continually saying/doing the wrong thing. (Baldwin and Costley, 2016, p.490)

Autistic girls have been considered to have less severe social and communicative behaviours than autistic boys at a young age, although some of this may be due to the invisibility of difficulties when masked by camouflaging behaviours. However, as adolescents and adults, girls have more social difficulties, particularly with peer relationships (McLennan *et al.*, 1993). The prevailing view is that the peer activities commonly engaged in by girls and women are more socially and communication dependent, compared with boys, whose relationships remain largely topic- or activity-based (sport, special interests) and who, as a result, often have fewer verbal and non-verbal interpretation requirements. Some girls prefer the company of males as they share more interests and do not engage in so many emotions-based conversations (Tierney *et al.*, 2016). Autistic author Rudy Simone describes this change in her own comparative social skills:

> I had many friends [...] until adolescence. All at once, my idiosyncrasies became very uncool, almost overnight. My social *deficits*, which prior to that point had just been *differences*, became glaring holes in my persona. (Simone, 2010, p.28 [Rudy's italics])

> [She is] not interested in talking with you unless it is about something she is interested in; [she] talks at length about her favourite subjects without checking if the other person is interested. (Parent)

There is very often a desire to make friends, but frequent rejection can lead to feelings of ambivalence and that it is just too much hard work (Tierney *et al.*, 2016). Stories of trying hard to fit in – and failing – were frequent in the responses. There was study, mimicry and effort involved to solve the social puzzle and gain entry into the arena of inclusion and acceptance. Liane Holliday Willey describes her own 'assimilating behaviours' which more recently have been termed as camouflaging and masking:

> I was uncanny in my ability to copy accents, vocal inflections, facial expressions, hand movements, gaits and tiny gestures. It was as if I became the person I was emulating. (Holliday Willey, 2014, p.29)

> People often got offended or bothered if they realized that I quoted a character from *The Vampire Diaries*, for instance, in a serious conversation or perceived me to be less authentic because of it. If I was rewatching some of my favourite TV shows or movies with friends and a character said the phrase I'd previously quoted, they'd say 'Wait, did you get that line from a movie? So they weren't your words?' and I wouldn't know what

> they meant because no words are my words: I didn't make up the English language or the rules about how to string together sentence structure.

> My voice can sound harsh and monotone if I'm not concentrating on making it sound nice.

Other difficulties arose not only from failing to understand the signals and rules governing teenage friendships, but also from the impact of making another person the object of a special interest and becoming unusually fascinated by and focused on them. The young autistic woman may seek exclusivity with the 'friend' and be confused as to why he/she would want to spend time with anyone else.

> I thought that Connie was beautiful and so clever to be able to play the piano. I followed her everywhere, and it was difficult to understand why she wanted me to go away at times, or why she wanted to be with other children and not me. (Lawson, 2000, p.58)

As they get older, most autistic girls perceive themselves as 'different' (Holliday Willey, 2001; Stewart, 2012), perhaps when comparing themselves directly with the social profiles of their same-gender peers. Many of the women in my sample did not receive a diagnosis until many years later, yet still recall this awareness.

> I feel like I have a different operating system [with] a very good emulator running on top of it. The few people I tell are shocked to find I'm autistic. I can fit in, I can behave like others up to a point, but it isn't me and doesn't fulfil anything within me. It's empty and meaningless.

> I was very aware that I was 'different' and didn't fit in, and I had no wish to fit in as I couldn't see what was so great about being NT [neurotypical]. I felt rejected as my attempts to bond with

> peers frequently failed, and I felt like my parents were ashamed of me as they thought I was weird and an embarrassment.

> The reward for trying hard to be normal was to be ignored because you were acting normal, and I look at stories online of kids who were going off the rails and I think, I should have just burned more cars. (Bargiela *et al.*, 2016, p.3286)

What also comes across from some of these women is a paradox that many autistic people seem to struggle with: a contempt for the superficial content of the relationships of their peers, coupled with a desire to be accepted by those same peers. In the responses, there is also the relief that has come later in their adult years that they no longer have to be part of this teenage world that seemed so alien. It seems that the teenage years bring all the stress and confusion of mature social relationships but none of the adult choices of being able to opt out (due to having to endure school).

On being told by his father to 'make friends' with a girl he had introduced her to, Wenn Lawson (at that time presenting as female) describes his strategy:

> She asked me lots of questions and to most of them I replied 'yes'. It seemed the safest thing to do; in my experience, when one answered 'yes' people were happier. (Lawson, 2000, p.17)

> I made a lot of efforts to fit in, but they all failed and by the time I was in my late teens, I'd given up. I'd known I was different since very early childhood. To be honest, these days I care very little about fitting in. I see the NT world and culture for what it is, and I have little interest in selling out to be a part of it.

> I tried to wear the right clothes or be interested in things others were, to fit in, but I never quite pulled it off. It's a bit like trying to speak another language that I'm not fluent in – I can get by for so long, but eventually I'm always found out and my ignorance is revealed.

Opinions on social relationships, particularly with other girls, are a clear indicator that these young women thought and felt differently to their peers. They had different agendas, different interests and different requirements from a friendship. Some were bullied, some were excluded and some were permitted to exist on the fringes. It is also the case that their peers were aware of their differences when adults around them were not (Bargiela *et al.*, 2016).

> Girls in real life are not something I enjoy being near, especially loud, squealy, hair-and-make-up high-schoolers.

> When I was being bullied, I was told not to antagonise these girls and actually I was only antagonising them by being myself. (Bargiela *et al.*, 2016, p.3286)

> One time aged 13 a girl did an experiment on me by calling me a bitch. I was confused because she was one of the few who was normally nice to me, or at least not horrid, and then she said, 'You don't know how to react do you?' She'd clearly noticed that I simply did not have a response in my repertoire to such things.

Others seemed not to rankle and engender the displeasure of their female peers, either by being invisible and/or of no interest, or by being endearing and tolerated to some degree.

> As a teen I was quite lucky – I was 'allowed' to hang onto the edges of two girls who had been best friends since they were young.

The additional expectations of young autistic women in terms of social ability, self-care, education and independence may lead to more visible mental health difficulties during this time. Peer rejection and loneliness lead more autistic females to be referred for professional support than autistic male counterparts (Tierney *et al.*, 2016). They may develop obvious signs of anxiety, self-harm or eating disorders, which may not be linked with autism by professionals as this may not have been diagnosed yet. Some of these behaviours can be incorrectly attributed simply to puberty and treated in a way that does not address the underlying stress involved in living as an autistic person in a non-autistic social world.

> As a teenager and young adult, I did what was expected of me in order to fit in. I went to night clubs, which I hated. I went to [Girlguide] camp, which made me ill as I was so distressed. Even after that I went on holiday to Spain with a school friend just because it was the expected thing to do. I came home halfway through and spent about a year recovering as my mental health was affected so badly.

Adult relationships

> Somebody asked me recently if there might not be some way in which I could enjoy doing social things. How about, he said, if we removed the pressure of expectations (to react, to talk) and kept the number of people to two or three and didn't get noisy, etc., etc. Well, I answered, if you took away all the things that make me not like socializing, I guess the answer is, yes, I might like that kind of social *activity*. (Kearns Miller, 2003, p.239)

> I sometimes feel as though I struggle with getting a good balance or reciprocity in friendships/relationships. I often feel as though I take more than I give in friendships, and that I give more than I take in romantic relationships. I can be quite all-or-nothing in that I dive straight in at the deep end with relationships. I can get very excited, very quickly, often imaging how we could integrate into one another's lives more fully.

Friendships and people interactions continue to be a major source of analysis, effort and anxiety for adult autistic women. Adulthood for some brings a greater degree of self-acceptance and awareness of the types of people and interactions that work best. The trying, difficult teenage years are left behind, and real choices about who to spend one's time with arise. The issues with friends are three-fold: first is the matter of identifying who might become a potential friend and knowing when they have become one; second is the actual social effort and understanding required to physically spend time in their presence; and third is the understanding of how the friendship needs to be maintained (through contact) in between meetings. All of these factors affect the ability of autistic women to make and keep friends and to tolerate the presence of other people to ensure long-term social contact; all are also directly attributable to the core diagnostic criteria of autism.

> Before the diagnosis I'd thought I had no friends because I was unpleasant; then I learned that it was simply difficult for me to communicate in the way that makes people comfortable forming bonds of friendship. Before the diagnosis, when I 'withdrew' it had always been attributed to me being 'moody' or 'sulky', when actually, inside, I often felt calm and happy and was surprised when people were angry. It explained why I had difficulty functioning in a typical way and found day-to-day life such a challenge.

> I see the way some of my acquaintances act towards other friends of theirs and they seem to have this [...] give-and-take/back-and-forth sort of interaction which looks totally effortless.

The issue of friends is a complex one throughout life for these autistic women, and it takes many years to get their heads around either what it means to be a friend or how to be around people without anxiety and fear of rejection and social failure. All those years of childhood feelings of difference take their toll and leave their mark.

> Still not sure what that really means, what it takes to be a friend.

> I remember a man at university saying to me, 'You know, Rebecca, you have to be a friend to have friends'. I was shocked by him saying so and still remember it strongly now – still wondering what I wasn't doing to be friend-like.

Personally, I have about five people that I make any contact with outside my immediate family (partner and children). They are all diagnosed autistic, have considerable autistic traits, or are gay. I do not have any neurotypical (NT) female or straight male friends; these two groups are too socially complicated and frightening for me to cope with (gay men are safer because the potential misread/missed attraction issue is removed). I make virtually no contact with these people unless it is to arrange a meeting or discuss a specific point or question. I do not miss their company and would probably not notice much if I never saw any of them again, even though I really like them and care about their well-being. The number of people I have felt a genuine 'rapport' with during my life is in single figures.

The frequency of interactions and number of people in the women's lives were typically small. They tended to meet on a one-to-one and fairly intermittent basis. For most, this was enough to meet their social requirements. For one woman, her partner was the only person she needed in her life. The quality of their relationship provided her with what most autistic women are looking for: acceptance without judgement.

> I never meet up with friends and have no desire to. My best friend is my husband; he truly accepts me for me. He has held my hand without judgement for the last ten years and I love him so much.

Interactions were reported to be exhausting, requiring both preparation and post-meeting respite. Women describe their awareness of personas and scripts to help get them through essential interactions with the outside world.

> It kind of feels like you're an outsider looking in and like there's this world that you're just kind of observing from the outside, and when you have to get directly involved in it, it can be a bit hard sometimes. (Milner *et al*., 2019, p.2398)

> Every social encounter requires constant decoding and then selection of an appropriate response. I have preprogrammed/learned behaviours for church, meals, restaurants, casual, semi-casual, formal situations. (Kearns Miller, 2003, p.255)

> One lady has produced a guidance sheet for interacting with people on public transport. She had listed how many times one should smile at the driver in order to avoid 'making a fool of oneself'. She explained that reviewing social interactions and analysing them in order to identify where things went wrong takes up a huge amount of her time and, of course, this is exhausting. (ASD specialist support worker)

What we can learn from these women is that large social networks are not the norm and that crafting a social world that fits within the autism is the best path to well-being. If autistic women can understand that their 'failure' to procure a large group of friends is actually perfectly typical, I hope this will lead to a greater sense of self-worth and acceptance.

> For me, even interacting with friends I've known for years is difficult. I have to make a conscious effort to sort of 'keep on task' when I am with a friend. So, in the end, I am exhausted and just can't face seeing them again anytime soon.

> When it's my turn to return dinner invitations, I invite eight to ten at a time, to repay as many invitations as possible at one time.

> I would say there are only three people I see once every few months, and I consider them to be my friends. Yet, even with them I feel like now, somewhat, we have not much to say to each other.

> My best friend lives in New York, and I usually see her [a] couple of times a year and chat to her on the phone or online/text about once a week. Recently, she's been visiting more often, and this has been a bit of a problem. I don't know how to tell her I don't want to see her so much without offending her, but I find her visits very tiring.

For some there was a sense that seeing other people 'got in the way' of them doing their own preferred activities. This, I would argue, is in direct contrast to most NT women who would choose socializing and companionship over solo pursuits.

> I have some other friends who I see occasionally, perhaps once every two months. This suits me fine as I find people hard work, and I simply don't have the time and energy to spend it socializing when there're other things I need to do.

For some of the women, their social interactions had to have some purpose or function; the idea of simply meeting others to chat held no appeal. It is commonly considered that sharing interests is a core facet of autistic relationships, and these women are no different in that respect. There was a sense of the relationship being on their terms and needing to meet their requirements, rather than for the purpose of establishing a mutual, empathic and emotional bond, in most cases.

> I don't want more friends really. That would be too much to take on [...] I suppose ideally I'd like a friend who was knowledgeable about IT and would give me free IT help, but that is the only addition I would consider making.

> I can be a 'user' in friendships: I like people who know more about things than I do, so I make an effort to befriend people who are clever and know things. I have a very low tolerance for people I perceive as stupid.

> My friendships are more based on a mutual exchange of knowledge and/or practical help or advice. We don't do 'small talk' or meet for a coffee for no apparent reason. All interactions have a purpose. I suppose some might say we're just using each other, but I think even NT friendships do that to some extent as NTs crave companionship just for the sake of it.

Some women have identified that there are particular types of people either who appear to be drawn to them, or whom they are attracted to.

> I think there is a kind of maternal woman who tends to take me under her wing – could it be the same type of woman who likes to 'fix' men? The problem with that kind of woman is that they eventually end up bossing me around or using me for their purposes. And when I find out, it is too late; and generally, what I have done several times in my life is just walk away without an explanation.

> I have one female friend as an adult who I have been friends with for over 20 years. It is likely she is also on the spectrum [...] With hindsight I think many of my male friends were probably Aspies too [...] They were all eccentric, colourful characters who were really interesting to be with.

As with their teenage selves, autistic women still find other women are not their natural peer group once they reach adulthood, with one study of clinicians noting that peer relationships with NT females were rare in autistic women seeking diagnosis (Cumin *et al.*, 2022). NTal women may be more socially adept and emotionally driven with an expectation of intuitive mind-reading or empathy for their experiences. Autistic women are often pragmatic creatures, quick with advice and solutions and less comfortable with a hug and a platitude. They may struggle to connect emotionally to the experiences of others due to an emotional delay in processing, a complete disconnect or because they don't share the same perspective about what matters and what doesn't. For example, an autistic woman may be extremely distressed by a point of injustice which would not concern an NT woman; an NT woman may be more concerned by a perceived social hierarchical sleight which the autistic woman would not have even noticed. The notion of empathy works both ways and arguably is difficult to achieve when each party comes from a different world view.

> I dislike other females; they are complicated and often boring. They rarely have the same interests and certainly not to the same degree. They gossip, judge people and talk crap a lot of the time. They put importance on things that don't matter, like what someone wears, looks like, social status, etc. They can be competitive, jealous and bitchy.

Online relationships

For autistic women today, the Internet appears to offer a space for developing friendships based on interests and not requiring the complexities of face-to-face interaction – no one cares if you're not wearing the right clothes or not making the right facial expressions. Some younger women said that all of their interactions were Internet-based and that they had no in-person social contact at all. Video-gaming was important to several of the respondents, and their involvement in these communities had provided them with friends. This suits many autistic people as it means that they can remain in the stress-free environment of their own home, while having contact with the outside world on their own terms – it's easier to log off than to remove yourself from an awkward party scenario.

> I have friends on the Internet. They are a mix of male and female, and points in-between. I talk to them on a varying basis, always one to one. I would like more friends, but I do not wish to burden them.

> Currently, I have many friends on Facebook, and for me this is an

> ideal medium as it saves me the awkward personal interactions. Yet sometimes I feel very lonely, with nothing but counsellors, advocates and a very distant – I mean real distance here – couple of siblings to hear me when I'm frustrated.

With regard to social media such as Facebook, Robyn Steward (Jansen and Rombout, 2014) talks about the confusion that can arise for an autistic person with the concept of 'friends' on Facebook:

> On Facebook you can unfriend a person. A lot of people on the autistic spectrum can become upset about this. They may ask themselves: someone is not my friend anymore? But a Facebook friend is not the same as a real friend. A real friend is someone who cares about you. They don't unfriend you. (Jansen and Rombout, 2014, p.66)

Animals

People aren't the only candidates to be potential friends for autistic women: animals featured strongly in the lives of some women and are generally understood to be important in the lives of many autistic people. Animals are easy to read (limited facial expressions), non-judgemental, unconditional and loyal, and have limited and easy-to-meet demands (food, stroke, walk, sleep). It is clear why autistic people often prefer animals to humans and feel that they have a real connection with them – perhaps operating cognitively in a more straightforward 'animal' way without agendas and deceit themselves.

> I like animals more than I like people. I've always said if I meet ten dogs I'm likely to get on with 9/10; the reverse is true with people [...] I've always felt animals understand me better than people and they make fewer demands on me. I prefer my dog to my best friend.

> [...] Animals. They are what I consider my true friends. I do

> indeed feel like I have a natural affinity to them, since a very tender age. I feel like I'm better able to read them than humans [...] Sometimes I do wish I were an animal, or at the very least someone who was 'as one with the wild', such as in some tribal communities, and lived a simpler yet inevitably more physically taxing life.

Alone by preference

Not every autistic woman feels the need for social relationships; some are quite happy being alone, having the freedom to follow their own schedule and their own interests. Home is definitely a sanctuary for many women – a place where they can leave the persona and internal social monitor at the door and relax. Twenty-seven per cent of autistic women preferred their own company, in comparison to 10 per cent of autistic men. Females (19%) were also less likely than males (40%) to state that romantic relationships were a priority for them in the future (Baldwin and Costley, 2016).

Leaving home can feel like an effort, a foray into hostile territory, and therefore some women can be in danger of getting 'stuck' in their safe place and rarely venturing out. This is fine if it is someone's genuine choice, but professionals need to be aware that she may need some encouragement to take a chance on the world beyond her walls.

> I like the way it's okay nowadays for people to just sit in a coffee shop by themselves. There's something nice about feeling you're part of the world and not having the stress of having to be communicating. (National Autistic Society, 2013a)

> I don't really feel lost without 'friends'; I don't feel like they're a requirement. It's just that it seems the right thing to do to get along in life in a more neurotypical fashion, which is almost a requirement as I can't escape it.

> I still struggle sometimes with things like phoning up to order

> a take-away; I'm very grateful that modern technology means I can order food without having to deal with a human being.

> I'm happiest when I don't have to leave the house or see anyone.

Social isolation

> *[I] have this incredibly strong, almost addictive, like, drive to be by myself and yet feel this, like, enormously crushing loneliness at the same time.*
>
> Kock *et al.* (2019, p.15)

Loneliness and isolation were mentioned by some women, who often found it a struggle to find like-minded companions as they got older. This was particularly the case if they did not have a long-term partner or children. This is not the same as seeking alone-time – either for preference or as a coping strategy for overwhelm or autistic burnout, discussed further in Chapter 13.

Joining groups and initiating contact with neighbours or work colleagues are simply not possible for some women – they feel intense anxiety about such things and perhaps would not even know where to begin. I know myself that I have jettisoned many evening classes and activities (French, kick-boxing) because the social requirements of the classes were too stressful and excruciating for me to contend with, despite being quite proficient at the actual skill being taught. Trying and not being able to maintain connections may feel like a bigger failure than not trying at all.

> Social isolation is not just about having mates to socialize with. It's true that if I go to the cinema, I go alone. I eat alone. I go on holiday alone and when I get home, everything is exactly how I left it. But it is more profound than that. If I am ill, no-one will bring soup or take me to the hospital. At the end of a working day, there is no-one to talk to about the stresses or the highs. If

> I am anxious, I stay anxious. I have no friends I can call to cheer me up. (National Autistic Society, 2013a)

> At this point in my life, I feel there is a total lack of friends to share interests, and that's not surprising considering my interests. I am a 43-year-old female with a very niche taste (within metal music there are several dozen subgenres and I care only about two or three of these).

Social impact of ageing

Seventy-three per cent of autistic adults over 55 years of age have three friends or fewer, with 65 per cent saying their main friends are their families or carers (National Autistic Society, 2013b). It has been suggested that autistic women may have less interest in marriage and children (Ingudomnukul *et al.*, 2007) and therefore we might conclude that more autistic women may age without families. We have also heard that autistic women have limited social networks and experience anxiety in social situations. These factors potentially lead to even greater isolation than is experienced by other older people. It is necessary to recognize that being older does not eliminate the features of autism, and socializing at any age will be difficult for these women, despite well-meaning invitations to day centres and lunch clubs.

> Left to my own devices I will interact very little and not build relationships, but I am aware that I risk a very lonely old age if that continues. It's easy to get set in my ways and not seek others' company as I get older, but I do want to try and have some worthwhile relationships during the rest of my life.

> The older I get the more lonely it feels as the people who really genuinely cared for me have gone [...] It's easier to stay home than make plans to go out, especially if it involves other people. We have our set activities and are comfortable in our own home.

> I suppose I should be afraid of isolation. It's never pleasant, and I hated it when I was younger before I married. However, if you change the word from 'isolation' to 'time by myself' it sounds quite appealing.

Despite continuing difficulties and social anxieties, my overall perception from my reading and experiences leads me to believe that adult autistic women often reach a place of self-acceptance as they get older, but that a sense of loneliness can often pervade. They are clearer about who they feel they want to spend time with, how often and how long for. They appear to be more comfortable with who they are, more aware of their limitations and more able to assert themselves to meet their own needs in social relationships. For some, it seems that the 'price' of certain friendships is not worth the social inclusion on offer and this realization is a sign of empowerment and self-value. Considering the time and energy spent by these women in attempting to fit in during their teens, it is encouraging to discover that there may come a time when they stop, think and realize that their own path is the right way after all.

Chapter 7

GENDER IDENTITY AND SEXUALITY

> *I didn't identify as either a boy or a girl (even though intellectually, I knew I was female). I identified more as an android or alien as I didn't believe I could possibly be a human as I was too different from my peers and could see things and see truths about life that they couldn't.*
>
> Autistic female

Gender identity

Studies increasingly recognize a link between so-called gender dysphoria (GD) and autism, finding that in comparison to typical children, autistic children are over four times more likely to have experience of differences in their gender identity (Hisle-Gorman *et al.*, 2019) and that 20 per cent of those with GD are autistic. This effect continues through adolescence and into adulthood (van der Miesen *et al.*, 2018). In adolescence, more birth-assigned girls experienced gender dysphoria than boys, but this was not the case in adulthood. Over-representation of autism in individuals with GD is seen frequently in research (Glidden *et al.*, 2015; Heylens *et al.*, 2018), but no one hypothesis on the cause is suggested; more likely it will be several (van der Miesen *et al.*, 2016).

For the purposes of clarity, 'sex' is used to describe biological attributes assigned at birth. 'Gender' refers to socially constructed attributes.

As an older autistic female, the vocabulary and awareness of anything other than a binary gender identity didn't exist for me and many of my peers when growing up, so we are late to the party on this. For myself, it would have been extremely helpful to have known that I was not alone in my sense of not feeling female as a teenager, particularly. I dressed as male, mimicked my male peers and was more of a son than a daughter. Most people thought I was a boy, and I am still frequently mistaken for a man despite having long hair and large breasts. I have always thought that there was just something undefinably 'male' about me that others can subconsciously detect. I made Airfix models and wanted to be a Harrier jump jet pilot, had my own woodworking tools and collected model cars, which in the 1970s was uncommon for a girl. I was considered an honorary boy at school and permitted to join in with 'bundles' (a popular 1970s playground game at my junior school which involved children throwing themselves on top of each other in a large pile and then trying to get out from under the pile). To be fair, none of the girls actually wanted to join in, so it wasn't much of an accolade. I would most certainly have identified as non-binary had such a word been available to me, and it would likely have been a great relief. Young, autistic and non-binary/trans young women have the opportunity to access communities of their peers and hence feel less alone or strange and relieve the potential mental distress that these feelings can bring.

Some research suggests that girls and autistic women may have a more masculinized or androgynous neurological profile (Baron-Cohen, 2002; Bejerot *et al.*, 2012) due to possible differences in prenatal androgens (Auyeung *et al.*, 2009). It is important to consider that the outward presentation of clothing or toy choice does not necessarily represent the internal cognitive profile. Some autistic girls wear pink and play with dolls, but their brain and thought processes tend to be more pragmatic, logical and less socially intuitive than typically expected of a neurotypical female.

> I hated the colour pink with a passion. I wanted to be a plumber when I grew up. Sadly this was frowned upon. I think I probably would have made a good plumber and earned a good wage.

> I don't feel girly, but I can do my act, and I would never want to be a princess. I'd rather be a superhero or action man!

Of those participating for this book, more than 75 per cent felt that they did not specifically identify with behaviours typically associated with girls, even at a young age. This was reported both by parents of girls and by adult women, but as mentioned above, it tends to be viewed diametrically, as either male or female, when in fact it may be simply a more gender-neutral behaviour. The majority of respondents used the word 'tomboy' (this word was deliberately not used in the question and was offered by the participants themselves). For those who didn't have a preference for typically boyish behaviour, they identified with something more androgynous:

> I was a tomboy, did not get into make-up, but wished I could be more like the other girls. I loved motorbikes, got one and learned how to take it apart and fix it.

> I was very much a tomboy when I was growing up, preferring to play with boys rather than girls. The nicknames my family called me when I was a child were 'dirty knees' and 'monkey' because I was either scrabbling around in dirt or climbing trees. I played with Lego and Meccano rather than dolls, and at secondary school in the 1980s, I took options in woodwork and metalwork instead of cooking and sewing.

> I related to boys easier, and I had more fun with them. Sometimes I would wish I was a boy; it all seemed so much easier for them. I never understood girls.

> [...] Not tomboy. Very girly, but do have logical and pragmatic brain. Not very emotional: like steady, even dispositions. Don't like games and drama. Hate pink; prefer blue and red, or navy and white.

> I'm no good at being a girl. (Milner *et al.*, 2019, p.2395)

> I am a heterosexual cis-woman. However, I found it very difficult to present as female growing up in the 1980s; I sometimes got my hair cut at the barber's and for a long time only felt comfortable in non-descript, baggy men's clothes. My attempts to 'pass' as 'one of the girls' were awkward and so I often tried to act and speak like a boy, even wearing the boys' clothes, even though I didn't want to be one... I think that trying to present as either feminine or masculine were both forms of autistic masking for me personally, and that I wasn't very good at either!

We have mentioned the 'tomboy' profile commonly seen in autistic women, and heard girls and women talk about their difficulties in fitting in with their female peers throughout childhood and adulthood. We've discussed how many are unable to identify with all things 'girly' and have a more typically masculinized, straightforward communication style. It should come as no surprise then that when trying to define her sexual and gender identity, the logical mind of an autistic woman can sometimes struggle to make sense of where she fits, who she is and who she might want to sleep with (if anyone). This sense of identity may not feel like it comes naturally and intuitively and may have to be 'worked out'.

> From 15 to 24 or so, I don't think I ever wanted to be a man, but I did really struggle with what seemed to be the expectations of me as a female. And I wondered at some points if I'd been born in the wrong-sexed body. I couldn't see myself in the women I knew or a future for myself. I had no sense of what my adult identity could be. I could not make sense of gender and spent some active years in the feminist and gender/sexual politics world.

> As an adult I do not think I perceive myself as a female. Although I know I am a middle-aged woman, and I am not a lesbian, deep inside I often perceive myself as a young man.

It must be stressed that confusion is not the case for all autistic women; some have a clear and strong sense of their gender and sexuality, regardless of their experiences with peers. However, it does seem like a higher percentage than would be expected find themselves perplexed and alone in their feelings that they are different from anybody else out there – male or female. It is also important to distinguish gender identity from sexuality, as the two do not necessarily correlate: for example, a woman who feels more male than female is not necessarily gay, or indeed transgender. She may be a happily heterosexual female.

> [...] Think more like a man: sensible, logical, even-tempered, no-nonsense, emotionally-level. Enjoy all things feminine, womanly (make-up, hairstyles, clothes, nailcare, grooming, decoration, cooking).

> I don't really understand the 'gender identity' concept; I have always felt female and been proud of it. I don't see gender as having an influence on my life outside of the physical/biological aspects: the differences between me and my brother relate to chromosomes, reproductive organs, inherent strength/height and the ability to gestate a child.

> I've never been a 'feminine person'. I've always been a little bit aggressive, I can't stand wearing make-up, I barely brush my hair. I go through phases where I feel like I *should* be more feminine because I'm embarrassed to be around people who are. Femininity has always been this missing piece for me, so I copy the women around me in order to fit in. (Schembari, 2023)

Women I speak to do not always define themselves in terms of neurotypical (NT), dichotomous labels of gender identity, sometimes preferring broader gender labels, such as 'genderfluid' or 'third sex'. This demonstrates the sense of not feeling either male or female, but something else. Studies in this area have identified similar findings (Kallitsounaki *et al.*, 2021; van der Miesen *et al.*, 2016).

Although individuals who define themselves in this way exist in the general population, it is among autistic females that I come across it the most. Other authors (Holliday Willey, 2014; Lawson, 2000; Simone, 2010) have also discussed gender identity in autistic women and found a more fluid sense of belonging.

> I define myself as a woman, but I am queer. I have always been queer, but the terminology to describe this didn't exist when I was a young person. It has never been an issue for me what gender other people were. I find people attractive based on who they are, not what they are.

> I very rarely feel like a woman. I feel like a man most of the time, but sometimes feel in-between, or neither, or both.

> [On being a woman] It's a malady I was unfortunately cursed with. I don't identify with my physical vessel in the slightest. I only see it in terms of how it pleases men; and I like being the cruel tease for fun, to snub them I suppose. It's like a tool. I think that's the simplest way to describe it. A vessel that I use to interface with the world around me, or at least try to.

> I came out as bi/queer at 18. At 48 I identify as binary/queer. I am about to start micro-dosing with T (testosterone)... I guess I never understood gender and why it exists. I am pansexual and these constructions are just meaningless. Just like many constructs. And perhaps constructs in general are something autistic folks question... My gender doesn't matter. I think it is that simple. However, on another level, if it doesn't matter why micro-dose T? I can't 100 per cent answer that. Except to say I feel like my voice should be lower and that would feel more comfortable to me.

> I have often debated whether or not I am transgender in the typical female-to-male sense, but the term 'gender fluid' fits a lot more.

In Chapter 1, we discussed the work of Baron-Cohen, Ingudomnukul, Bejerot, Auyeung and colleagues, who all suggest that testosterone plays a part in the development and profile of autism. This leads to the conclusion (by some) that women on the autism spectrum present a less feminized profile. This has typically been interpreted as meaning that autistic girls are more masculinized. As previously discussed, Bejerot *et al.* (2012) suggest that the profile may simply be more androgynous (i.e. non-gender-specific) as opposed to specifically masculine.

> When I say I don't feel like a woman, people are likely to assume that I mean I feel like a man. I don't. Never have. Nor do I feel alienated by my body, its female shape, its female cycles. (Kearns Miller, 2003, p.157)

> I still see myself as relatively genderless, as I did when I was much younger. I have traits derived from both sexes, but I don't fully identify with either one. It's only safe to say I lean more strongly towards masculinity than I do femininity. There has been talk of 'third genders' emerging. I feel like I'm one of them; akin to the *hijras* of India. In layman terms I feel like a chimera.

> I do not feel either. I am glad to be a woman, merely because it gives me the ability to have children, which I love. I don't feel especially female, whatever that is; indeed, I have always preferred the company of men. I feel more comfortable when in a social setting with men, which is probably why I coped very well working in a prison surrounded by 1700 men.

> I don't feel like a 'woman'. I just feel like a 'thing', other and alien.

This androgynous profile is described by women themselves as more masculine – perhaps for want of a better word when considering something like gender, which is typically believed to be dichotomous.

> I remember saying many times during my teens that I wanted to be male in my next life. This was because their lives seemed

> more interesting, and it seemed that they got a better deal in life. It was not really that I wanted to be male, more that I got on with them better and felt alienated from females; and also being female meant boobs and periods, smells and moods!

> She chooses to wear masculine clothes because it's so much simpler, she doesn't have to worry about the intricacies of make-up and things. (Milner *et al.*, 2019, p.2395)

> As far as I can recollect, I have always perceived myself as a male. I cannot really describe what it is about me that makes me think I'm a guy and not a woman. It's like my inner voice is a young man. The moments when I am most at peace and enjoying myself (i.e. walking alone listening to music on my headphones), those moments I am a young man. I don't think I'm very feminine in my gestures or my intonation. I know I walk like a man too.

> When I pondered on the act of sex, I often felt like it was more fun from the male's perspective. Being the girl seemed boring, like a chore, rendering oneself as an object for the time being. And orgasms? I snorted at the thought of them, thinking them the stuff of myths; and I still do, having never managed one myself. I guess I'm going to come across as brutally honest here, but I enjoy the thought of male-on-male sexual encounters in my mind. They excited me more than heterosexual interactions. In my dreams, come to think of it, I am almost always a male entity. Perhaps I really do have a secret want for being male.

Transgender and autistic

> I feel a euphoria in being seen as who I really am.

> A lot of people give transwomen a hard time about their

> appearance or even existence. With autism, insults and criticism cut straight to the bone every time. Please keep that stuff to yourself. We're trying very hard and just want to be normal like everyone else.

Transgender and gender-diverse individuals are between three and six times more likely to be autistic than cis-gendered individuals (Warrier *et al.*, 2020). This study reviewed five large data sets comprising of over 640,000 individuals. Transgender people scored higher on systemizing, sensory sensitivity and lower empathy using self-report measures. This suggests not only that are transgender people more likely to be autistic, but also that there may be many undiagnosed autistic people within the trans and gender-diverse communities. In adulthood, 11.4 per cent of those experiencing gender identity differences are autistic compared with 3 to 5 per cent of the general population (van der Miesen *et al.*, 2018).

Despite the number of women who described their more male gender identity, the only transgender people who responded to my requests for participants were transwomen – male-to-female transgender people. I had no responses from cis-gender females now living as men although one cis-woman was due to begin taking testosterone supplements without the intention of fully transitioning. However, I was able to speak to Wenn Lawson, an autistic psychologist, writer, researcher, poet and academic, who has made the decision to transition from a female to a male gender identity. He told me that a psychiatrist he had spoken with had said that he had known of some autistic people who had transitioned and had lost their diagnosis along the way; they were able to live and function so well in their 'new' gender (with the social requirements associated with that gender) that they no longer met the autism criteria (Lawson, 2014). For Wenn, there is a distinct difference between feeling not female and feeling that you are actually male. We must remember that diversity across autistic people is as broad as in any other population and that not all autistic women who do not relate to typical female experience necessarily want to actually change their physical gender.

> I am one of those people who, while not feeling female, have never felt that I am actually male.

De Vries *et al.* (2010) studied a group of young people referred to a gender identity clinic and found that 7.8 per cent of these individuals met the criteria for autism spectrum disorder (ASD). Pohl *et al.* (2014) found that autistic women show a greater tendency for 'gender dysphoria' and 'transsexualism' than NT controls. On being asked why they thought that there were more transpeople within the autism community, two participants had these comments:

> Maybe because autistic people aren't influenced by others and are more likely to just be themselves. That's my best guess.

> I already had a sense of alienation being autistic. I can't relate to other people, and this has allowed me to take a step back and assess who I am. I had already taken one step back being autistic; this (identifying as trans) was just another step back.

Anecdotally, it is widely believed that there is a higher proportion of transgender people within the autism population than elsewhere, both trans men (female to male) and trans women (male to female). One adult Asperger syndrome service in Brighton reports that 9 per cent of their 170 members identify as transgender, the majority being trans women. They also report that at the time of first contact with the service almost all of the trans people who approached them for support were undiagnosed autistic. Many stated that their gender identity issues had masked their autism. On asking those within the transgender community, I've been told anecdotally that autism is very common, although usually undiagnosed. My own experience of working with individuals with both autism and gender identity confusion leads me to believe that there is a connection between the two.

> There's certainly a connection between my autism and my transgender/homosexual stuff. They're part of my neurotype that

> makes me, me. I don't think they can be separated [...] As far as if I'd only had one issue or the other: if I didn't have autism, I feel I would have transitioned in my late teens. I wouldn't have let a little bad news tell me not to do it. I would have also been more self-sufficient (I never held a job for more than three months back before my diagnosis with autism). If I'd just been autistic, I really worry I would have been one of those people commonly referred to as 'neck beards' or 'men's rights'. By being female, but having to live as male, I learned to understand both genders and their ways of thinking (typically). I really value that insight, now.

The strong sense of not belonging with one's same-sex peers and feeling alienated from one's birth gender is common for autistic people. Therefore it is not surprising to me that many individuals feel that their brain and body are so incongruent that they are unable to continue living within the 'wrong' body. I believe it is important to support individuals in understanding both aspects of who they are in order to achieve positive outcomes and manage expectations. Changing gender/sex will not alter many of the challenges that an autistic individual may face and will not be the answer for some. For others, it is exactly the right choice.

> It was less about being called towards one thing (living as a female), more being pushed away from the other thing (living as a male). It felt like the correct course of action... I didn't change anything; I was always like this.

One man I worked with had long-standing gender identity issues that were causing him enormous depression, anxiety and suicidal feelings. He was conflicted about whether to transition and tormented by uncertainty. He was then diagnosed as autistic. Prior to this he had believed that gender identity was the all-encompassing challenge affecting everything else in his life (work, relationships, mental health, sexuality), but later he came to see that being autistic was the main factor and that his gender identity could be explained for him by the cognitive and psychological impacts of being autistic. He had previously been trying to find a place for himself on a binary NT gender/sexuality spectrum of either male or female. I suggested to him that maybe the autistic gender/sexuality spectrum was different – more androgynous, less dichotomous, more fluid – and that his error had been to attempt to categorize himself using a system that did not apply to him. He found this reframing helpful and was able to make a decision to continue to live as man while accepting and expressing his more androgynous/feminized profile privately and on his own terms. For each person, the right path will be their own, but they may need support in finding it.

> The big reason behind all this is so I can be comfortable in my skin. I've only recently started to understand how much more normal I can feel like this. I assumed all of my anxiety and awkwardness was due to my autism, but it turns out that gender was a big part of those problems, too.

> I put on a high-pitched, breathy female voice and lift the intonation depending on my level of comfort. I naturally slide into it. As soon as I realize someone is the same brand of weird as I am, my voice tone lowers, and I show my true self... I have learned that all trans people experience impostor syndrome: What if the problem is me? What if I am faking it? But why would I?

When asked when they first had a sense of difference in terms of their gender identity, the transwomen's responses indicated that this came early in their lives – perhaps even before any awareness of their autism.

> Eight is when I noticed it, but I didn't understand what it was until high school. I just didn't feel like a boy and felt disconnected from my body and felt parts of it were wrong. I have always had a very feminine personality also.

> I was 11 years old and at a music festival with my mum. I looked to the right and saw a group of boys playing football, or whatever. I turned to my mum and said: 'I don't think I'm one of those'.

> [...] Around puberty, 13-ish? When I saw all the girls going through a puberty that I wasn't, it just felt so wrong. I had some idea earlier, but I wasn't sure why. I always tried to play with the girls at recess but was always shunned. I never understood why.

For many trans people, the decision to come out and transition is a difficult one, perhaps made more so by their autism. Often their fears were largely unfounded, and support was forthcoming.

> The biggest impact was from my tendency to take everything at face value. The few documentaries I saw about transgender women always showed their lives falling apart and them facing tons of discrimination. Because of that, I hid my feelings so deep no one had any idea. It wasn't until my early 30s that I'd finally heard so much positive about being trans that I was comfortable coming out and transitioning. Of course, my family and friends all accepted me, and my wife even helped me with all the things I needed help learning. Hell, she even married me while I was fully presenting as female, and we were both in dresses. I really wish I'd known then what I know now, but I trusted the handful of things I saw to be honest about it.

In working with any autistic person of any age, it is necessary to include gender identity in any discussion on the impact of their autism. Women find great relief in knowing that their sense of not belonging in terms of gender is also part of being autistic. It means they are not alone or at fault; it's just part of the autism deal. Supporting autistic women to accept their identity and not continuously compare themselves unfavourably with NT women or men, or dislike the less typically female or male aspects of themselves, hugely increases confidence and self-esteem. Finding resources, videos and support from other autistic women to foster a sense of belonging and community is more valuable than can possibly be imagined. An opportunity to be open about gender confusion without judgement is necessary for these individuals. Any support must also begin with the autistic starting point, rather than from an NT perspective, which may be very different. Where a person feels strongly that they are transgender, support should address both autism and transgender issues and needs.

> I had no style as a male. I am now interested in fashion. I didn't go through all this to not show it off. My friends were always female. I have been able to make friends more easily and my experience has also made me more open-minded.

Sexuality

It has been suggested that autistic females have a greater propensity to be asexual, gay or bisexual than would be expected within the NT population (Ingudomnukul *et al.*, 2007). Autistic women specifically are found to 'show a significantly lower degree of heterosexuality when compared to autistic males' (Gilmour, Melike Schalomon and Smith, 2012, p.313). In Dewinter, De Graaf and Begeer's research (2017) more autistic women were found to be in same-sex relationships than typically developing women. Others (e.g. Pohl *et al.*, 2014) find similar outcomes. Within the women questioned for this book, only around 50 per cent defined themselves as heterosexual. My experience suggests that some autistic people can have a more blank-canvas approach to sexuality and that some decide on a pragmatic basis what their sexual preference is, rather than it feeling like an innate part of who they are. My own sexuality is something I have never felt the need to define. Evidence would suggest that I am heterosexual, yet when I'm asked, I have a tendency to reply in a characteristically autistic fashion, that as I haven't met every person in existence, I can't possibly know. There may be a woman/trans-person/other who might sweep me off my feet, but I haven't met them yet. I have always been baffled by the certainty that most NT people appear to have around their sexuality. How can they be so sure?

> The short answer is: I'm a lesbian. But since questioning where the borderline is between male and female is my bread and butter, what it means to be attracted to women is a bit of a slippery concept. I'm open-minded about having sexual partners who are androgynous/have different gender identities/have penises, so basically, I can be attracted to anyone with breasts and no facial hair.

> I always knew I had feelings for women, but this never seemed a realistic thing for me: I had never met a lesbian. I was 26 when I first got with a woman, and I haven't looked back since. I was never confused by my sexuality really; coming out wasn't a big deal, perhaps because I did it so late and these days most people aren't bigoted about it. Several friends had worked it out long before I did. I think I spent a long time barking up the wrong tree because that's what was expected of me, and I had a series of failed relationships with men because I was aspiring to be a conventional woman; I was trying to conform to what society expected from me.

> Queer is the most accurate; sexuality is a spectrum, and it has shifted and changed throughout my lifespan. I regarded myself as bisexual for many years, but in new terminology I would be demisexual or possibly asexual aromantic at this point in my life.

> Primarily heterosexual although not always, and I only want to have intimate relationships with someone I am comfortable with emotionally. I guess sapiosexual [sexual attraction to intelligence] is close or perhaps demisexual or both!

> I don't feel like a woman in a sexual sense. I am not a lesbian and have gone as far as experimenting to see whether I was. I have kissed two girls, in one very drunk night, and enjoyed it as much

> or more than kissing a man – girls don't have scratchy beards. I have also dated a lesbian girl, got as far as having dinner and a car ride, and was revolted when she touched my leg. So that is how I know I am not a lesbian. Plus, I have this idea that a proper family requires a male and a female, so that children get the right exposure to both genders as role models.

> I wonder if my sexuality is due to my autism, as I was vulnerable as a teenager and males took advantage. But I'm not sure I would be gay if I had better skills to deal with sex and relationships.

Asexuality

One study has found that autistic individuals show a higher rate of asexuality compared with NT controls (Gilmour *et al.*, 2012); again, due to difficulties with social interaction, a preference for solo activities, sensory issues with intimacy and a different perspective on gender identity, this should come as no surprise. Around 20 per cent of the women I spoke to defined themselves as asexual. Most had felt that heterosexual relationships were something they were supposed to have and enjoy; therefore, most had attempted to have these before eventually learning that it was okay not to want or like such intimate engagement.

> I was born without sexual feelings. Nobody's going to have a non-sexual relationship – everyone has sexual feelings. I'm in the minority. (Kock *et al.*, 2019, p.12)

> I think my aromantic identity has been more fluid over the years, and certainly when I was in my 20s and desperate to fit in with my peers, having a romantic partner was something I believed would give me that acceptance and approval I needed.

> I just felt like a female that wasn't that interested in relationships. I never felt gay or anything. Just more interested in my hobbies

> and having fun in life than in romantic relationships. I always felt pressure though to be like other women and have a boyfriend and as though I was a bit of a failure because I didn't want that.

> I feel sexless. I don't like sex [...] I never have wanted to have sex, ever. I did it because I thought I had to.

For some, the realization that being asexual was an acceptable way to be came as a great relief, having previously assumed that there was something either psychologically or physically wrong with them for not seeking a relationship.

> At age 51, I became aware that the term 'asexual' was not just a description concerning amoebas (as I'd been taught in biology) but also a valid sexual orientation. After extensive reading of forums, blogs and a lot of honest soul-searching about my past failed attempts at dating and relationships, I realized that the description of asexuality as being someone who does not experience sexual attraction fitted me perfectly. To know that there was a reason for my lack of sexual attraction to other people was a huge relief, as was discovering a whole community of people online who felt the same way as well.

> I obviously wasn't normal and felt too ashamed to tell anyone for fear of them rejecting me as being too weird. I persevered with trying to mend myself by reading even more magazines and self-help books and experimenting with having sex both drunk and sober, but nothing seemed to work. I concluded that I must be the dreaded f-word, frigid, and spent years feeling broken, worthless and consumed with self-hate.

I think the keys to a happier life are awareness and acceptance (both self- and society's) of people's differences, combined with knowledge and self-understanding. If both autism and the whole spectrum of sexuality are discussed openly and sincerely in mainstream society, then maybe there will be more tolerance of people's differences, and this will lead to young people having the courage to be proud of who they are and not feeling so much pressure to conform.

Chapter 8

PERSONAL RELATIONSHIPS

> *The biggest kind of thing that would affect our relationship in the beginning is that if he was talking to me and I saw a dog, I would, like, completely blank him out and just be all consumed by the [dog]...he used to really get upset.*
>
> Kock *et al.* (2019, p.14)

> *Relationships are still so demanding, so confusing. I want to relate to other people but I'm not sure I can survive the pain of it all. Some days my brain is so sore from trying to work out what it is I am supposed to do or to say, that I just cannot do it for very long.*
>
> Lawson (2000, p.97)

For autistic women, personal relationships are as fraught with confusion and uncertainty as any other social interaction. Additionally, these usually include emotional involvement, intimate physical contact and sharing one's time, space and possessions for extended periods. Societal gender expectations lead us to believe that women are good at this stuff, that nurturing and caring come naturally and intuitively and that women who find this tough are somehow cold, damaged or just plain 'weird'. As well as all the autistic reasons that make finding, establishing and maintaining a relationship with a significant other difficult, by adulthood, autistic women have had the message hammered home that they are not ideal companions.

We have heard how these women mask and hide in order to present a more acceptable public version of themselves.

> When you are seeing somebody about once a week and he lives about 40 miles away from here, you can kind of present a sanitised version of yourself, you could rein it in. (Kock *et al.*, 2019, p.16)

A close personal relationship is a place where a person ought to be able to be their true self: their best and worst self, accepted without judgement. To reveal this real self to a partner is terrifying and makes the woman vulnerable to further rejection. She may also not be a great judge of character and therefore end up making a poor choice of partner, perhaps feeling grateful that they would even bother with her defective self. The majority of autistic women seem to want a partner, with or without the sexual element, and only a few choose to remain happily single.

Reading signals

The autistic profile makes reading both verbal and non-verbal social signals tricky, and this is no more evident than in the sphere of personal relationships where it is all about the subtlety, the flirtation, the unsaid. For an autistic woman this is a minefield of misunderstanding and uncertainty, which can lead to obsessive stalking-type behaviour or, alternatively, vulnerability to abuse. She cannot tell who is interested in her, or who is not. If you cannot read people's desires and intentions, things become very stressful and sometimes dangerous.

> Due to the autism I missed a lot of social signals and had no idea if or when someone was attracted to me. I didn't understand the rules of dating, despite having by now graduated to *Cosmopolitan* magazine and using it as an instruction manual for my socializing; and to be honest, I couldn't see the point of playing games anyway.

> I'm told that when younger, my inability to read signals left a small succession of men feeling rebuffed and vaguely puzzled. I'm flattered and bemused. I hope they were good-looking. Some years ago, I was in a relationship. He had to practically club me over the head and drag me into the cave before I realised he was interested. (National Autistic Society, 2013a)

The communication style of an autistic woman can be blunt and to the point. If she wants to know if someone wants to have sex with her, she may ask them outright before even knowing their name. Alternatively, she may waste no time in telling them that she will not be having sex with them, even before they know hers. One woman interrogated potential partners on the first date, wanting to know everything about them and their relationship history. She had no judgement about their responses but felt that by knowing this data about them, she was better able to predict how she needed to behave and to better predict their responses. This is not how the dance of attraction is supposed to go. The intrigue, the uncertainty and the anticipation are all part of the fun for neurotypical (NT) people; not so for the autistic woman. She just wants to know.

On many occasions I have been described by male partners as 'too heavy' for asking for their thoughts on how they thought the relationship would proceed – to be fair, this was sometimes on the second date. This was assumed by the men to be a sign of somewhat premature emotional attachment, which scared them. In fact, it was simply a need to know exactly what it was; I didn't mind either way, I just wanted to know. The concept of 'going with flow' and 'seeing what happens', favoured by many, was too stressful and uncertain for me.

Selecting partners

Autistic women are pragmatic creatures and may have more practical requirements from a mate, whose needs they will have to meet and presence they will have to tolerate. Sharing interests and lifestyle were important considerations for the women I questioned. Undoubtedly, concepts of 'chemistry' and 'connection' apply to autistic women when selecting partners, but this is not something that anyone mentioned.

> I chose my husband because he had some amazing gym equipment I wanted to use. (Hendrickx, 2008, p.24)

> He had an interest in virtually all of my favourite activities, even my favourite pastime that no one else had ever expressed an interest in. (Hendrickx, 2008, p.24)

Some women described their partners as needing to be part-carer and to look after them, as they felt unable to manage alone.

> Before the bizarre rush to acquire a mate, the thought of being alone didn't bother me in the slightest; if anything, that made me feel empowered, like I didn't need anyone and I was a free spirit. Since after the event, and now, it's the total opposite. I question my likelihood of survival without another mate. It's not due to the craving of emotions either: no, it's just I realize more and more how inept I am at taking care of myself and at life as an entirety.

> I like having a partner, as long as they are able to help me with things. Essentially, they have to be a bit of a carer for me, too, as well as a partner [...] I like having a partner but could never live with anyone. I need my own space and don't like feeling pressured or to have to be social or compromise all of the time.

> I have never lived on my own for more than a few months as I really struggle, but I manage okay with a live-in partner. I have paid help with housework.

Sensory preferences may form part of the choice of a partner, which are separate from physical attraction in the typical sense.

> Sometimes all I need to keep from falling over the edge is to look at Tom's face. I am stunned by the looks of his face, not so much because he is an attractive man, but more because, in the structure of his face, [I] see so many of the visual elements that appeal to me – linear lines, symmetry, straightness, perfect alignments [...] It is a visual respite for me. I am oddly calmed when I look at his features, so calmed that I find just looking at him puts me at ease. (Holliday Willey, 2014, p.95)

As expected from a lifetime of negative responses, some women did not feel worthy of having any selection criteria for a partner and were willing to go out with anyone who asked. Some described their partner choices as 'random', which is not surprising – if reading people, 'connecting' and understanding one's own emotions and those of others are all difficult or impossible to do, partner selection becomes almost a lucky-dip approach. Just like crossing roads or assessing danger, without context such decision-making is problematic.

> For a very long time I believed I was a hopeless case. 'How could anyone love me?' I just wanted one person to walk beside me and accept me for who I was. (Hendrickx, 2008, p.88)

> My boyfriends tended to choose me, rather than the other way around, and I was just grateful that someone thought [of] me [as] girlfriend material.

> I had absolutely no interest whatsoever [in having a boyfriend] during my teens. I'd grow incensed at the sight of public displays of affection, seeing it as a waste of time and a needless distraction of focus. I only started feeling a sudden desperation when I was about 22 [...] I was rather abruptly consumed by thoughts that my life would never achieve fruition if I didn't have a significant other for support. Looking back at it now, I wish I never let that feeling get the better of me [...] It's left me broken and torn.

Potential partner as intense interest

At many points in my life, I have engaged in borderline stalking of selected people whom I have become infatuated with – thinking about them constantly, wanting to know everything about them, what they did and where they were, and planning how to accidentally 'bump' into them in the hope that they would be as pleased to see me as I was to see them. As a teenager, I used to cut my arms, and this sometimes involved etching a boy's name into my skin with a safety pin. Once I showed one of these boys what I had done, thinking he would appreciate my handiwork and recognize my devotion to him. He was horrified and thought I was quite scary and mentally unwell. He wasn't even my boyfriend: he was just the latest target for my obsession. Thirty years later, the scars are still visible. I remember surreptitiously picking up a discarded cigarette end dropped by one object of my intense adoration, along with a coin he had given me, and storing them lovingly in a drawer in my room. I am only grateful that Facebook didn't exist in my teenage years – I would have been worse.

> After chasing him obsessively for months, he finally rebuked me in an angry, frightened voice, 'You're not a girl; I don't know what you are'. That was the first time I realised I could scare people, but I still couldn't fathom what I'd done wrong. (Simone, 2010, p.80)

> If I fancied someone, I would get totally obsessed with them to the point of not enjoying life. I would sit by the phone for hours, waiting for them to ring. I would pace around the house all day with nothing in my head [but] that very person. It was well beyond the usual infatuation.

The focus of intense interest on people – rather than objects, as often typified by autistic males – has been noted previously and, along with the desire to belong, it should be of no surprise that some autistic women become deeply obsessed with another human. Autistic women cannot read the signals of interest and attraction and may struggle to perceive how the other person is feeling, which might not be as they wish.

> Of course, it's important to consider others, but all I could feel was my own need. I still find it difficult to put myself 'in the other person's shoes'. I can only feel my needs and myself – everything outside is foreign and alien to me. (Lawson, 2000, p.113)

Autistic women may need support to understand these strong feelings for another person and learn how to put them in perspective and recognize that the other person may not feel the same way. A friend or mentor may need to explicitly state what socially acceptable behaviour is and what may be considered scary and weird.

Staying single

Some autistic women I spoke to had never had a personal or sexual relationship, and others had tried (usually because they thought they were supposed to) but decided that it wasn't for them. For some this was related to being asexual but for others simply a choice.

> [...] Relationships where it's all equal and you look after each other – I'm not very good at looking after someone else, I'm afraid. So, no it wouldn't work. (Kock *et al.*, 2019, p.16)

> I never had friends to come up to my flat or small get-togethers and now I am quite fearful of people coming to visit me. I never met a boyfriend either but I have now accepted that I will always be single and am happy living on my own. (National Autistic Society, 2013a)

For others, the lack of relationship was more troubling, and they would have liked to have found a partner, but for various reasons this had not happened. Kock *et al.* (2019) found that most autistic women wanted to be in a relationship. It may be that they had missed signs of attraction or had not felt strong attraction to anyone themselves. What is known is that gender, sexuality and libido may be experienced differently for autistic people and that norms in these areas should not be applied. The biggest issue for the women who had no established relationships was often a feeling of failure in an NT sense: that they had not managed to achieve what other people had in terms of finding someone who chose them as their exclusive partner. This is a very visible aspect of adult life – people around you know if you are single. Being single is often viewed negatively in our society: 'no one loves you, therefore you are unlovable'. We know that autistic women want to fit in, be accepted and be invisible. For some, not having a partner is the ultimate sign to the world that you are just no good.

> Quiet men are usually attracted to me as they see me as caring. I have never found any Asperger guy attractive, which is sad, but again I feel as though anyone who I would feel confident talking to would depend on me to talk for them. I've no idea why I feel this way; but I would have had plenty of opportunities for boyfriends, but they just didn't attract me, and I didn't feel it was right to pretend that I fancied them when I didn't.

> I have never had [a boyfriend] and used to feel a freak because of this. Men would pick up that I was nervous of them and probably still do. I still feel a freak to be honest.

For trans autistic people, living in a body that does not reflect their inner self, combined with the usual suspects of autism, may result in a reluctance to have a relationship.

> I've never been in a relationship – partly because of lack of social skills when I was at school and lack of contact with women since then (due to hanging out in the autistic community so much), and partly because I don't want a sexual relationship until I've finished my sex change, and I've got a body that I can be proud of.

First sexual encounters

The range of numbers of sexual encounters reported by the women I spoke to spread from zero to more than 30. Earliest sexual experiences were at 14 years of age, and many involved alcohol and some regret. A sense of gratitude that anyone would choose them, wanting to feel 'normal' plus, sadly, sometimes some naivety and coercion, can lead young autistic women into sexual encounters that are less than positive. Young autistic women are in great need of support in learning the rules of the NT world and in building self-esteem *vis-à-vis* a world that views them as different.

> As a teenager, I thought that if someone wanted to have sex with me then it meant that they liked me. I felt intensely proud that anyone would pick me to want to have sex with. I had no idea that for many young men, there wasn't much of a selection process, and my willingness was all that was required. I also didn't say 'no' because I didn't know I was allowed to. I thought people wouldn't like me if I said 'no', and I wasn't going to risk that.

> It was quite exciting discovering sex. I remember using the phrase 'I did that!' after giving him an erection.

> I had sex for the first time when I was 16, and it was part out of curiosity and part coerced by my sexual partner. I regretted that first experience then and still regret it now. He was such an idiot, and I didn't feel anything special, other than dirty and embarrassed.

Vulnerability to sexual assault

> I'm prey in a world of predators. (Milner *et al.*, 2019, p.2397)

The notion that girls and autistic women are particularly at risk from predatory individuals is well reported (Attwood, 2007; Holliday Willey, 2012, 2014). Misreading cues, naivety and taking what others say and do at face value can all lead to problems, particularly for a vulnerable woman. More than 50 per cent of participants reported sexual abuse in one study (Bargiela *et al.*, 2016). Autistic women are several times more likely to experience sexual assault and domestic violence than their neurotypical peers, and many experience multiple incidents (Sedgewick, 2018). They note difficulties in interpreting the motives of others and lack a peer group with whom to get guidance or assess whether a person's behaviour is within the range of acceptable or normal.

In one study (Cazalis *et al.*, 2022), nine out of ten autistic women reported sexual victimization with over 75 per cent of participants having experienced multiple events. Two-thirds were aged 15 years or younger when first assaulted. Autistic women believe what they are told and assume that other people have good intent because they themselves do. Women in my sample described themselves as 'gullible', 'vulnerable' and 'naive', and many women I have worked with report being taken advantage of, exploited and assaulted.

The known characteristics of autism can result in serious danger when applied to sexual situations. Many of the women I spoke to reported multiple occasions where they had been abused, attacked and/or raped. If you cannot determine on an individual basis who is safe and who may be a danger, due to being unable to intuitively pick up the signals and read the context of the situation, you are left with two choices: trust everyone or trust no one.

> As a young woman, and because of my inability to understand social context, I was in real danger on a number of occasions; one of them in particular could have ended very badly for me. I trusted him completely and took his word like the gospel; he could've spirited me away to just about anywhere and my mind would be absent of any ill intent present. I was obsessed by his countenance, at what I took to be at face value, which was probably completely the wrong impression.

> I've been in a couple of abusive relationships. I'd describe most of my exes as not very nice people, but then I guess that's why

> they're exes. I'm not sure I'm a good judge of character. I think I've been obsessed by people and been blind to their faults.

Sadly, it does not surprise me that autistic women could be more vulnerable to rape and serious sexual attack. An inability to read and assess people and situations can clearly lead to dangerous and distressing consequences. I have often remarked that I am amazed to have made it this far without ending up in a ditch due to the many poor decisions I have made, which could have ended badly through my misreading or failing to spot others' hidden agendas. I suspect that there are many women who have been subjected to this kind of situation but feel too ashamed to tell anyone what happened because it would have perhaps appeared so obvious to their listener. It is hard to explain why you thought something was a perfectly good idea at the time, only realizing your mistake after the event – and being aware that other people would judge you for making the choice you did.

> My first experiences were not willing. I lost my virginity at age 14 to my cousin [after suffering a] rape. I misread cues and ended up in situations where dates expected sex and I froze and could not fight them. I got pregnant at age 16 as a result of one of those encounters. (Hendrickx, 2008, p.82)

What I have found interesting is the way that some autistic women have been able to get over traumatic, personally invasive events, such as sexual attack. While rape is undoubtedly harmful both mentally and physically, and nothing must detract from that, it does appear that some autistic women are able to see the event quite objectively and move on from it. It goes without saying that each individual's experience and perception will be different and should be supported according to their individual experience and needs. One autistic woman describes her experience of rape and how it sits in terms of other stressors in her life.

> Once I was raped. But this actually ranks very low in my list of

> stressful life events (so much so, that I've never bothered to mention it in any of my counselling sessions over the [years]). It happened because of my social naiveté [...] When I realised rape was inevitable, I shifted goal to simply staying alive. Thus it was with a sense of relief rather than trauma that I survived this incident [...] On the other hand, a type of incident high up on my stress list involves the difficulties of communicating with co-workers. I am still as helpless as ever at dealing with this sort of thing. (Kearns Miller, 2003, p.243)

Liane Holliday Willey (2012) recalls a number of incidents of sexual assault that occurred due to her naivety. She talks about needing to carry out 'cognitive restructuring' to understand and look at the events in a more positive way. I use a similar approach using basic cognitive behavioural therapy (CBT) techniques, which can be found online and in CBT books. I am loath to recommend anything specific as different people favour different approaches, although for me as a practitioner and for personal understanding, I have yet to find anything as well written as *Cognitive Behavioural Therapy for Adult Asperger Syndrome* (Gaus, 2007), along with its companion workbook *Living Well on the Spectrum* (Gaus, 2011).

Other women describe ways in which they have learned to protect themselves following difficult experiences with potential partners.

> I listed ten qualities I wanted in a man. Sounds strict, but I had to set limits for myself to keep from being vulnerable.

> Life has not led me to think that my own feelings and emotions are valid or meaningful, so I use others as a yardstick for knowing what is acceptable.

Sex and intimacy

In my previous book on sex and relationships in autism spectrum disorder (ASD) (Hendrickx, 2008) I noted that autistic women were more likely to see the emotional and physical side of sexual interaction as separated from each other than was generally expected in NT women. Often their perspective was closer to what is usually perceived as a more male approach to sex – pragmatic and not always requiring emotional intimacy. Many of the women questioned for this book expressed similar thoughts. For some, the presence of a partner for meeting sexual needs wasn't required at all.

> Libido was like an itch that needed scratching, and the most effective method would be to satisfy it myself by masturbation. The connection here with my autistic traits I feel is that interacting with another human requires more effort (also more stress and anxiety) and the outcome is not as predictable as going solo, as it were. Obviously, there is also my requirement for space and solitude, and if sexual satisfaction is all that is required at that time, then why complicate matters by involving someone else?

> Like the sensory sensitivity kind of things...skin against skin could be quite unpleasant...sometimes trying to put a sheet or pillow between me and the other person...and it gets kind of interpreted as a sort of rejection...or just I think probably what bothered me a bit more was the idea that they thought I was weird. (Kock *et al.*, 2019, p.13)

Women reported confusion about the concept of intimacy and emotional connection. Some said that they didn't feel it at all, and others felt it very strongly but not necessarily in relation to physical sex.

> For me, sex feels like a tangible, concrete way to connect with my partner.

> I don't know that I understand the concept of emotional closeness – it's too vague, too abstract – but physical closeness is a means of feeling safe with someone when at your most

> vulnerable and most 'naked' self, which I think, for me, is as good as it can get.

> I am still very confused about the connection between intimacy and love. I tend to view sex as a basic animal instinct, a need that has to be satisfied, like hunger or sleep. When I have sex with my husband, I do not like to think of him as my husband, the person I share my life with, and who I have a child with.

> What the body needs and what the spirit needs are different at different times. (Hendrickx, 2008, p.90)

> I am not capable of telling if the other person has an emotional attachment to me or not, but as long as I do then sex can proceed. (Hendrickx, 2008, p.91)

The sense of 'connection' for some women did not come from sexual interaction, but from companionship and intellectual sharing – something more mentally nourishing, rather than physically so.

> Having sex with a person I love does not make me want to connect on an emotional level with him while I am having sex. It is as if sex is too functional, too dirty, and (why not?) a bit risible and over-dramatic, to smear it on someone I care for. I prefer the foreplay, kissing, hugging and caressing. And as for connection, I'd rather connect with my loved one through the mind, through sharing ideas and activities, and through comforting physical contact.

> I have to have some manner of bonding with the person before the thought even emerges about allowing that person access to my nether regions. The thing is, though, sex is not a priority; I could quite happily get through life with someone I genuinely liked without having sex. What I desire the most is mental mutuality. Once that is there everything else falls into place.

Successful relationships

Autistic women tend to form relationships either with other autistic people (Hendrickx, 2008; Simone, 2010) or with those far on the other end of the social and nurturing spectrum (teachers, nurses, counsellors, carers). In male/female relationships, the most common pattern is a double ASD partnership. In same-gender relationships, either extreme can apply. Whatever the combination, it is clear that autistic women find satisfying relationships, but that these can sometimes be unconventional by typical standards.

> I have been with my partner for two years. We met online and have yet to meet in person. It doesn't matter to me that we have not actually met. I describe being in love as feeling literally giddy, and I wonder how I got on before.

> (Following diagnosis) I now have my own bedroom after 22 years of marriage! It is not the death knell of our marriage – it is what we need. We have different body clocks – I am a night owl, my husband is an early riser. I sleep better now. I have my own space to decompress – being alone is so very important to me. It is recharging.

> I don't have a typical marriage: we are quite separate as people, we don't co-sleep or have an intimate relationship, but we are devoted to each other. It has sometimes been difficult for me to accept that this is what suits us both because of what society expects from adult relationships, and I have found myself questioning our choices and thinking 'but we should be doing this, or that'. I also have to be careful who I disclose this to because a counsellor recently presumed that my marriage was 'broken' because of our separateness, and this was very harmful.

> I once thought I was incapable of falling in love with someone and connecting the way that others seemed to. My partners were chosen at random. Just in the past two years I have learned that I am capable of forming a connection. Curiously enough this

> connection is with another individual who has AS. I wonder if that is part of what made it possible. (Hendrickx, 2008, p.47)

The partner is often the best friend and only person required in the woman's life and her relationship with them intense (Sedgewick, 2018). Her social and emotional needs may be fairly small (in comparison to an NT woman) and are most easily met by a partner with similar requirements. Autistic people may be attracted to her for the same reasons she is attracted to them: shared interests, intellectual knowledge and an appreciation for a direct and straightforward approach (no game-playing, no mind-reading). For autistic women, NT partners may be too socially complicated and emotionally demanding, expecting intuitive, empathic reading of emotions and requirements that are beyond them.

> You get to share [activities] with one another and it means that the world is twice as big, twice as colourful, twice as detailed... (Kock *et al.*, 2019, p.17)

> When it all works it's amazing and it feels great and I feel really good about myself; it's like 'look I have a personal connection to the other human being'. I can do it like everyone else can. I can have this like everyone else can. I am not that abnormal that I cannot form a simple connection to another person. I can do this! I imagine it's what winning the lottery feels like. (Kock *et al.*, 2019, p.17)

> My relationship is crucial to me; my partner is also my best friend and constant companion. I am loyal and faithful; I don't see any other male as attractive or of sexual interest when I am in a relationship. My partner feels like part of who I am. I don't miss him when we are apart – I can often forget about him completely when I'm busy at work. Neither of us knows when the other is wanting sex and neither knows how to initiate it, so we have somehow developed a routine to approaching it, which sounds boring, but it isn't; it totally works for us.

I have a belief in an intuitive ability that I call 'adar' (in reference to the reputed gay radar, 'gaydar', where gay people can spot another gay person), by which autistic individuals are drawn magnetically to each other without any conscious thought. My partner, Keith, and I met online. Neither of us knew that the other was autistic when we started to communicate, nor for several years afterwards. We are two peas in a pod, delighted to have found each other after many failed attempts. How on earth we managed to find each other, I don't know. I put it down to adar. We can happily spend 24 hours a day together for extended periods and not get irritated or overwhelmed (as is the case with every other human being in the world). As an autistic woman, this has been a once-in-a-lifetime experience for me, a respite from the performance I put on for the rest of the world, a place to truly call 'home'. I cannot emphasize strongly enough what a difference this has made to my life.

> I think my husband and I get along very well. I don't think I have ever had such an honest relationship as I have with him. With other partners I always felt as if I was acting. With him it is like taking my shoes off. When she first visited us, my mum was surprised as to how well we got along as a couple, considering we seem to interact so little.

> My husband is my rock; I really don't think I could go back to being on my own. I have become reliant on him to support me. I cannot believe that I coped for so long independently before I met him. I do believe that if he hadn't come into my life I would have committed suicide. The level of exhaustion I felt was awful. I sometimes wish that I had never met him, because not only have I trapped him, but I have trapped myself by having children who really need me.

A good partnership can provide an autistic woman with the acceptance and support to reach her potential in other areas of her life. Autistic women need support in recognizing a nurturing relationship and identifying what that looks like for them. It is important not to judge how people live and to support women to work out what they require to make a relationship manageable for them. Unconventional set-ups might be the answer for some: co-habiting might not work, sex might not be a requirement and separate rooms may be a necessity. Unconventional people require unconventional solutions to conventional arrangements. What is clear is that many autistic women are living happily in relationships with their partners and families.

Chapter 9

PREGNANCY AND PARENTING

Having a child is said to be an enriching experience for any parent. For me this enrichment came two-fold: as a woman, and as an autistic woman.

Autistic mother

Parenting as an autistic woman has, until recently, been a concept largely overlooked. Despite knowing that autism is an inherited condition, the assumption has perhaps been that – in line with the 'only males get autism' default – children were autistic as a result of their fathers' genetics alone, but we now know that this is not the case. The experience of caring for another human is difficult for most mothers, but when you throw in the challenges of coping with people, change and environmental stimuli, which autistic women can find overwhelming without a child in tow, life can get overwhelming. Children are, after all, people. Being autistic generally means that relationships with people are sometimes confusing and draining. It would be no surprise then to discover that autistic women would not want to be virtually attached to another person all day, every day for a number of years of her life, but that is not *always* the case. Regardless of the feelings involved in the decision to become a parent, autistic women need support for the duration of the journey. Parenting is not easy when you are neither socially intuitive nor flexible. Despite these challenges, 85 per cent of autistic mothers describe parenting as a rewarding (Pohl *et al.*,

2020) and largely joyful experience, and they feel intense closeness and connection to their children (Dugdale *et al.*, 2021).

> As an autistic woman, becoming a mum taught me an immense lesson in empathy, tolerance and care: a lesson in love. I learned that I can successfully ensure the survival and well-being of a creature who depends 100 per cent on me. Now I know what it is like to love someone, I can apply that to other people, and I can measure, I can classify, I can understand the process of love and what is involved. Being a mum has made my emotional life much, much richer, and much clearer. And knowing that I am an Aspie mum, who can empathize with her autistic child like no other mum could, makes me feel empowered, and confident that I can raise a happy human. And that is no mean feat.

> It's a great ongoing project that allows me to research things, obsess and shop online. I would say my baby is my new special interest.

> I was much more attuned to my children's needs, but sometimes too much that it physically hurt – I couldn't bear for them to feel that way so I would be a rescuer – which limited their opportunities for emotional growth at times. With my own therapy I have been able to separate my thoughts and feelings from theirs.

Wanting children

I have met many autistic women who have absolutely no desire to become a parent, as well as individuals who have been obsessed by the idea from an early age. Some of us take on this role more by accident than design. The concept of autistic women as mothers (often of children who also have autism) is largely overlooked by research, support and society in general. This is, I suppose, initially due to the 'only men get autism' viewpoint along with a perhaps mostly unspoken and maybe unconscious perspective that autistic people don't do relationships and wouldn't have children or be very good at taking caring of them. Around half of the women questioned for this book had children. Most had at least one autistic child and/or with other developmental conditions. Research has suggested that autistic women have a lower interest in marriage and children than neurotypical (NT) women (Ingudomnukul *et al.*, 2007), and this was certainly mentioned by some of the women in my sample.

> I never craved marriage or children and saw much female behaviour as silly and disempowering.

> [...] [No interest] whatsoever: maintained my entire life that I was not having children – even when we got married.

> I was never the little girl who wanted to have children. Even as an adult with children, it baffles me how anyone knows when they are ready to have them.

> I was 100 per cent sure that I didn't want children until my late 20s; then, when I met my (now) husband I knew with certainty that we would make a good parenting team.

> I initially didn't think I wanted children until I did. Then I really did, and nothing else mattered.

Others had a very strong yearning to have children for one reason or another.

> I always had a desire to have children. I wanted to be married and have five children. As I got older and not yet married, my number wished for got a little smaller [...] one of each sounded pretty good.

> Someone else to focus on. I hope it will make me less self-obsessed.

> I've always wanted to have a child but was always too afraid of childbirth itself growing up; and then after I was diagnosed, I was afraid that I wouldn't manage with the constant presence of another person, given how draining I find people.

Pregnancy

> [Pregnancy was] very planned, with military precision. I bought lots of things like [a] thermometer and ovulation test strips, and made a diary, and read up on the fastest way to get pregnant. It only took three months of trying.

Pregnancy is an exciting and overwhelming experience for any woman, but for an autistic woman, the experience may be somewhat more intense. She will have to cope with feeling completely out of control of her body, which changes almost by the day. She also has little control over the process that needs to be adhered to. There are appointments, new people and plenty of physical contact from strangers: both those needing to perform examinations and random strangers who feel that touching a pregnant women's stomach is acceptable behaviour. She may not have a social peer group of friends who are pregnant at the same time or have been previously. This can make this an isolating and frightening time, with no one to share worries with. Autistic mothers are more likely to experience both pre- and postnatal depression than non-autistic mothers.

> My sensory sensitivities took over, with even my own smell causing me to feel extremely nauseous.

> Pregnancy was terrorizing the first time. I was all of a sudden *afflicted* by pregnancy and therefore not the owner of my body any longer; nothing was within my control, and it was awful, just awful, not knowing how it would end.

> I have said in the past – to the horror of my listener – that pregnancy was the worst time of my life. It was really hard to see my body change shape so quickly. My usually dodgy balance and lack of spatial awareness made it very hard for me to move without knocking something over or falling or banging my limbs somewhere. The worst of it was, perhaps due to lack of social imagination, I didn't know whether at the end of the ordeal I was truly going to love my baby as everyone else seemed to think – I was too terrified of being judged so I kept my fear to myself.

> If I had had a full diagnosis – not just a suspicion – that I had AS [Asperger syndrome] when I got pregnant, perhaps the whole experience of spending ten long months of uncertainty, which led me to depression, would have been different.

Typically, some autistic women take on pregnancy as a special interest and devour every scrap of information that they can on the subject.

> It was very exciting to find out I was pregnant. I was looking forward to it all and scared at the same time. I wanted to know how to do everything. I read every (literally *every*) publication that I could find on what to do during pregnancy and how to take care of a baby and child. It was very helpful to take away my anxiety of doing everything right. I think, for the most part, I did know what I was doing. There was some confidence that came with all that reading.

Personally, I loved being pregnant because I liked being special, and it was easy to chat to people because they only wanted to talk about one subject – me and my expanding belly. I had horrendous morning sickness during both pregnancies but otherwise I was fit and healthy, stubbornly refusing to moderate my exertions and behaviour throughout. My son had to be induced after a particularly vigorous evening of dancing at a wedding made my waters break. I took my driving test at 36 weeks pregnant with my daughter and was still working as a lorry driver with my father at the time. I never felt in any way maternal or feminine.

> I would read books and needed to know what was happening at every stage of the pregnancy – how big they were, if they had fingernails, what their weight should be. The weight and height thing carried on after they were born, and I loved looking at the graph in their baby book to see what percentile they were on and got a sense of joy and satisfaction that they were above average – it felt like I was doing something right.

For those supporting autistic women through pregnancy, it is important to provide clear information about the processes that they will be expected to go through and also opportunities to ask questions. They may not have any peers who have been through the experience to talk to. When making a birth plan, consideration should be taken with regard to sensory issues, such as physical touch, pain thresholds and communication approaches.

> Asperger women report the need to feel more empowered about their birthing day and their experience is reliant on three factors including: clear communication, sensory adjustments and change management. (Autism Women Matter, 2013)

Giving birth

All of the information-gathering, mental and physical preparation and planning during pregnancy are the build-up to the actual giving birth. For the woman who prefers a schedule, the realization that giving birth quite frequently does not go to plan (despite her meticulous efforts) and that the process is likely to be out of her control – either by nature or medical intervention – is an utterly terrifying experience with no known end point. Autistic mothers were more likely to feel that the birth process had not been explained sufficiently to them (Pohl *et al.*, 2020).

> What is the purpose of a due date? I think you should have a due month, much less specific! When my due date came I sat at home waiting. Nothing happened and I became highly agitated and upset. I paced around the house wondering why nothing was happening [...] I couldn't process the fact that what was supposed to happen obviously wasn't going to. (Grant, in Hurley, 2014, p.66)

> After the delivery, I withdrew. I curled up into a ball and tried to comfort myself by sucking the roof of my mouth. The nursing staff left me alone and I slept on until the early hours of the next morning. When I awoke, I remembered I had a baby and I knew I needed to act like a mother or else I might lose him. (Lawson, 2000, p.80)

Autism Women Matter (AWM) (2013) conducted a survey with mothers on the autism spectrum and found that their birth experiences had been affected by the lack of support for their autistic needs. The whole experience of giving birth is extremely overwhelming for an autistic woman, who may feel completely terrified about the huge range of stimuli – both internal and external – that she is required to tolerate. It also may be the case that she does not behave in a way typically expected of a woman about to give birth. She may be particularly quiet because she doesn't know what she is expected to do or ask for, or alternatively she may be extremely distressed if touched, for example.

Autistic mothers describe feeling misunderstood by professionals and are more likely to end up in conflict with professionals than non-autistic peers. Eighty per cent of autistic mothers were worried that disclosure of their autism diagnosis would change the behaviour of professionals towards them (Pohl *et al.*, 2020).

> I was told to push again for next delivery; when I asked why, they said 'second baby' and laughed – they meant placenta, but I was terrified as I thought they meant twins. (Autism Women Matter, 2013)

> The main thing was that they didn't believe me when I said it was nearly time to give birth. I didn't make any noise and was so quiet going through contractions that they said I couldn't be anywhere near ready. When they checked, I was fully dilated and had to be taken straight down to the labour suite. (Autism Women Matter, 2013)

> People coming in and out of the room were disruptive. I ended up locking myself in the bathroom in the dark for eight hours of my labour. I had the same repetitive soothing music on for pretty much the whole labour. (Autism Women Matter, 2013)

> The ward was hell on earth. I can't sleep with strangers in the room so I was awake all night, and my baby screamed all night. None of the midwives helped me. I hated the noise, the chaos, plus my vomit phobia meant my anxiety levels were through the roof. (Autism Women Matter, 2013)

> They dimmed the lights for me and let me play the music I wanted, even though it was 80s pop instead of calm music. (Autism Women Matter, 2013)

> I had a home birth with two private midwives; I was well supported. I felt safer and more comfortable at home, rather than going to hospital with strangers and bright lights. I did a lot of research [...] I had my son by candlelight, my husband in the pool with me. Sensory wise I didn't want to be touched unless I asked for it; I also didn't want talking, and I had quiet music. (Autism Women Matter, 2013)

Breastfeeding

Autistic mothers are more likely to have difficulties producing an adequate milk supply, and other difficulties in breastfeeding were also reported (Pohl *et al.*, 2020). Infant feeding services are inaccessible and unsupportive to autistic mothers due to a lack of understanding and services which are not tailored to the mothers' needs. Becoming a mother was especially difficult for autistic women due to the changes in routines and lack of social support and sensory challenges added to the experience (Grant *et al.*, 2022). Experiences and feelings about breastfeeding varied in the women I spoke to.

> I loved having that time to just sit and be with my baby. It gave me the excuse to have time out from everyone and everything and just sit and be still with my child. (Autism Women Matter, 2013)

> My mum didn't breastfeed because she found it too painful. I am feeding my baby with expressed breast milk using a pump because we were unable to establish breastfeeding directly. My baby wouldn't latch on, and it was important to me that she had breast milk.

> I fed both of my children. I made it my life's duty. I fed my eldest for 3½ years and my youngest for 4½ years. That's eight years between them.

If a woman wishes to breastfeed she should be supported to do so, but she may need additional help in working out how she will manage sensory issues and in understanding her baby's needs if these are not obvious to her. She may need to ask many questions and be shown several times what to do. It should not be assumed that this understanding is implicitly or intuitively known as this may not be the case. It is important that she does not feel judged or a failure as a mother for not finding it easy. Guidelines suggested for supporting breastfeeding among women on the autism spectrum include:

- using visual instructions and diagrams
- direct verbal-communication approach
- avoiding innuendos and metaphors

- being aware that individual support may be preferable to breastfeeding groups
- verbalizing your intent to touch if needing to make physical contact
- considering reluctance to try a new approach as potentially temporary; the mother may need time and supplementary information in order to embrace changes. (Pelz-Sherman, 2014)

For those who choose not to breastfeed, equally they should not feel judged or guilty for not 'doing the best' for their baby. If it is simply too uncomfortable or stressful for a woman to feed her child, she may be doing more harm than good by persisting. The well-being of the mother generally best supports the well-being of the child.

Autistic parenting

> 'Why can't you be like other moms?' That hurt. I'd be singing opera very loudly in the car. Apparently other moms didn't do that. (Simone, 2010, p.140)

The experience of parenting is life-changing and all-encompassing for any woman. For an autistic woman, additional challenges arise. There are expectations for socializing her child, birthday parties, school meetings and playing, all of which mean not having much time to herself, which may be crucial to her functioning and well-being.

> [...] Truthfully? Loathsome, and with little return. Both my children have autism as well, and it's been grim – fighting for diagnoses, fighting for education, fighting with the LAs [local authorities] for provision, etc. It's like a constant fight that you can't back out of, and it never ends – it's always time for the next

> Annual Review or IEP [individualized education programme] meeting or Phase Transfer.

> Babies have round-the-clock needs. They're stressful, messy, unpredictable and demanding. Basically, they are everything that an autistic person finds hard to cope with. Gone was my precious alone-time. Gone were my carefully crafted routines. Even my body was no longer my own, transformed first by pregnancy then by postpartum hormones and breastfeeding. (Kim, in Hurley, 2014, p.26)

> The sound of my daughter crying was debilitating. I turned into a monster. I threw plates across the room and screamed 'shut the fuck up!' I didn't see mothers experiencing the level of rage and violence that I felt. I thought it must be because I am different. I tried to calm my rage through yoga and meditation, but nothing could calm the shutdown that I didn't know at the time was happening. Since my autism diagnosis, I don't yell. I learned I could stop it way earlier by using noise-cancelling headphones with white noise playing and separating myself from the sound of her crying. I tried to fix my parenting style and every time I failed at neurotypical strategies, I internalized that it was me that was the problem. (Schembari, 2023)

> It's so hard! My partner keeps saying he told me it would be hard, but there was no way to prepare me, no way to explain what it's like. I regretted it in the first few weeks after she was born because I thought I couldn't do it, but it's getting easier. I seem to be linked in with lots of support services now because I've been very open about how hard I'm finding it.

Many women writing on the subject of being an autistic parent describe feelings of inadequacy, and thinking that everyone else is doing a better job than they are. They report that parenting is an isolating experience, that they feel judged and unable to ask for support (Pohl *et al.*, 2020).

> I still feel the pangs of sheer inadequacy. My peculiarity will smash me in the face time and time again and I think 'What the hell am I doing raising kids? I'm no mother at all!' (Kearns Miller, 2003, p.195)

> Other mothers had more money, more patience, more stability and never seemed as stressed as me. They talked to each other in the playground, they met each other for coffee. I was never invited. (Simone, 2010, p.140)

> I often marvelled at these women that I knew who would go out in the evenings to shop or socialize or attend events with their children. I crashed. (Kearns Miller, 2003, p.215)

> Sensory issues made parenting small children difficult for me, particularly the food mess which comes with weaning toddlers – it makes me feel sick and uncomfortable.

> The crying! Oh, the crying and whinging! That was awful when they were little. It used to go right through me. I could cope if there was a legitimate reason but not when there wasn't.

> I was rubbish at playing make-pretend and found it so boring. Give me an activity such as baking, crafts, Lego sets, football, going on walks and little adventures; I was in my element and loved it, so this was all of our playtimes. Luckily, they weren't really interested in tea parties for the teddies or anything like that. I definitely lack the imagination to come up with elaborate stories.

> Playground pick-up was excruciating. I clicked with (what I would say now, were) other ND [neurodiverse] mums, but it was a horrible experience, meaning I would often be late to pick my kids up to avoid the experience.

> I used to find that I didn't know when my sensory cup was full, and then suddenly I couldn't cope, and I would get upset or

> angry. This would often confuse the children. Learning about my own diagnosis was crucial to changing this.

> I hope that, when I don't show my love for them in the more traditional ways that other parents do (it has been pointed out to me, for instance, that I seem to hug and interact with them less), they still recognize my love for them in qualities like the determination with which I stand behind them through thick and thin, like the fierce mother defending her young. (Kearns Miller, 2003, p.199)

Other mothers mention the intrusion and difficulty involved in tolerating their child's friends visiting the house, as having any person in their homes is something that many find a challenge, let alone a noisy, messy, irrational experience. The autistic mothers in my survey are often aware that their children have more to tolerate than their peers and are aware that they can come across as quite different to the parents of their peers. 'Coa', writing in *Women from Another Planet?*, compiles a list, from which the following are an abridged selection:

- mother with extra-embarrassing habits, such as lack of make-up, hairy legs and who is liable to appear in public still in bedroom slippers with pen in mouth
- mother who cannot model social skills (beyond her level, which they have surpassed)
- mother with annoying and unpredictable processing delays and requirements [...]
- mother who provides a largely asocial environment, with 'rarely anyone here besides us, because that's how I need it to cope' [...]
- mother who requires them to take on adult roles beyond their years. (Kearns Miller, 2003, p.203)

Other autistic writers talk about their sense of inadequacy:

> The parents I know seem to have the same kinds of experiences to recount and the same kinds of problems to relate. My worries and blunders come from places they do not seem to know exist [...] This used to bother me tremendously. It used to make me feel I was incapable of being an acceptable mom. (Holliday Willey, 2014, p.99)

> As my children grew older it became more difficult to cover up my sense of inadequacy. (Lawson, 2000, p.87)

There was also a commonly felt fear of being 'found out' as somehow incapable of caring for their children, which manifested in an even greater need for masking and not asking for help.

> The [disadvantage] that worries me is that perhaps somehow I could be seen as a worse mother if I officially have Asperger's; I know it doesn't make me any worse of a mother but I worry that somehow it could be used against me and I don't trust Social Services to understand Aspieness.

> I found the baby years excruciating. Looking back, I am sure I had postnatal depression. I remember having to fill out a form that checked for it and being so utterly convinced that if I answered truthfully my babies would be taken away from me. So, I lied and made out as though everything was fine, and because of this I didn't get the support I needed.

Some women expressed the idea of striving to be a 'good mum' and, in true autistic style, seeking to do this to unfeasibly high and unattainable standards. This combined with the sheer relentlessness of childcare led to them feeling that they were failing to be the parent they wanted for their children and being entirely depleted in the process of trying.

> On a good day, I think my daughter is lucky that I can 'see' her and 'hear' her. I don't force her to comply with social expectations. My

> autism diagnosis and experience have taught me that her needs are valid. I trust that she knows what she needs. But then on bad days I feel sad that my daughter got stuck with me for a mother. Once, at her preschool, my daughter had to fill out a Mother's Day survey with questions like, 'What's your mom's favourite thing to do?' Her answer was: 'Lie in bed'. I felt so ashamed that her answer wasn't something more exciting. I worry that I'm a low-energy parent and don't play as much as other parents. On days like that I feel I'm failing her. (Schembari, 2023)

> I love them dearly and they have kept me going when I wouldn't have bothered, but being what is expected as a 'good parent' has broken me in ways they will never know.

> I need a lot of alone-time to self-regulate – having small children, and thus very little alone-time, nearly broke me. I loved my daughters so much, and I didn't have the resources I needed to be the enthusiastic, fun mother that I wanted to be.

> Being a parent gave me a purpose and I have therefore done everything I possibly could for my children. It was my job to be the best mum I could be. I haven't always got it right, and when I think I have got it wrong, I feel it strongly and ruminate for weeks.

Some women feel that their autistic personality has provided them with positive abilities as a parent. It is likely that there may be a lot of reading involved with an autistic mum (Simone, 2010) – which should come as no surprise – as well as colouring, learning and 'doing' activities. Other women felt that their autism brought a positive sense of rightness to their abilities as a parent, which came over as a sense of pride and determination.

> As an autistic woman, I can focus on what is really important. I always put my kids as a priority in my life. I wanted them to have what they needed in material things and in their environment, like I did growing up.

> My own need for routine was very useful with small children: they got into sleep patterns fast and never got tired or hungry. It meant that our home life was pretty relaxed.

> [...] My determination to do it *right*, as is defined by myself.

> There is some advantage in having a mother who does not project her own needs and wants on her children, and who just accepts them for who they are. (Kearns Miller, 2003, p.212)

> I spent lots of time with the children. It was a very safe place to be. It did not matter whether I played games with them on the floor, did finger-painting, played with home-made playdough or joined in hide-and-seek; they never said I was dumb or stupid. (Lawson, 2000, p.85)

> I'm very organized because I have to be. I already use lots of lists and reminders, I'm good at sticking to a schedule; we always have food and nappies in the house.

Being mum to an autistic child

Given the genetic nature of autism, it is highly likely that autistic parents will produce autistic kids. Those autistic women who had an autistic child spoke of a special bond with that child and of having the intuition to know what their child needed even when it was different to what all the books and advice stated. They felt that the sharing of their diagnosis helped form a closer bond with their children and a more instinctive way of knowing what their children needed, and that they were able to translate and mediate for them to other people (Dugdale *et al.*, 2021).

> I never felt alienated from him. I never felt this abyss that many NT parents of autistic kids say they feel between them and their autistic child. (Kearns Miller, 2003, p.212)

> I love being able to really understand my kids.

> In Adrian's case, the books were wrong. Any baby care book that doesn't include the topic of over-stimulation is not credible. (Kearns Miller, 2003, p.195)

> I have a personal crusade to get kids who have certain social issues tested and, if relevant, diagnosed with autism. I don't understand the denial of certain parents; it makes me very angry. Perhaps this is even caused by my own faulty social imagination. Because as soon as I saw what I thought were signs of autism in my son, I had him diagnosed. I faced the facts, and I live with them; I don't understand denial.

Grandma is autistic

Being an autistic grandparent is a completely unresearched area. There may be expectations that women will fulfil a grandparent's role following decades of caring for their own children, when in fact they may be exhausted and wanting to spend time focusing on themselves. The assumption and expectation of women as willing and natural nurturers can rear its head again when considering the role of grandmother, and lead to further disappointment and guilt when Grandma is off and away kite-surfing (or long-distance cycling, kick-boxing and paint-balling, in my case).

> When my youngest child reached 18, I felt a very palpable sense of a weight being lifted. I know they still need me, but not every minute of every day. I have started to look forward now to a life for me without them. I'm glad I had them, but it was desperately hard, and no one knew.

> I am a much better granny than I was a mother. I can enjoy the good bits, but I don't have to worry about getting everything right for them – that is someone else's job. It allows me to be so much more relaxed than I was with my own kids.

In summary

Overall, we could summarize that autistic women make perfectly good mothers (and grandmothers), but often do things in their own unique style. It is perfectly possible for them to produce children who feel accepted, listened to and valued for who they are; children who are allowed to be independent and find their own way; children who accept difference. It would be interesting to study the children of autistic women and see if they follow any patterns – perhaps this style of parenting has advantages. For the majority of women, parenting doesn't appear to come naturally, but their way with logic, trial and error and commitment appears to compensate quite nicely.

> I certainly don't mother the way most women mother. My affect may still be flat as a pancake on too many occasions (though I've taught myself to smile more and laugh more and touch more), but I know something now. I think I do. Maybe I do. It appears likely that I'm a good mother, a loving mother. How very peculiar! (Kearns Miller, 2003, p.195)

Chapter 10

EDUCATION

> *My school guidance counsellor would call me into his office to raise concern on why I am always in the opposite direction of my peers. If everyone is at lunch then I'm in the classroom; if everyone is in the library for a class then I'm in the Early Years section of the library.*
>
> Autistic woman

At the risk of stating the obvious, a child spends a large proportion of their waking hours at school. School is not home. School does not have Mum/Dad/carer/family in it. Nor does it have a perfectly colour-coordinated, unplayed-with collection of My Little Ponies, or X-Men, for that matter. School has people in it: lots of them. As Rudy Simone puts it, 'Most of the Aspergirls said the same thing [...] school was boring and they were bullied' (2010, p.27).

For the child with a diagnosis of autism spectrum disorder (ASD) school constitutes a lack of control in all aspects of their world and hence can be a place of great trauma and anxiety. It is a constantly social environment with few places to hide or be alone (but you can bet that she has found all the hiding places that do exist). It can also be a place of knowledge, usefulness and structure. The extent to which the experience is positive or negative for the child is often a result of the understanding of her autistic nature by those in authority and their willingness to help her out. For girls, the aforementioned late or non-existent diagnosis and limited understanding of the female presentation ('She's quiet: she's fine') can mean that the school experience is often far from positive, as we shall hear. Eileen Riley-Hall, in her book *Parenting Girls on the Autism Spectrum* (2012), presents a whole chapter outlining education options and processes in both the US and the UK, which covers the practicalities and considerations with far more skill than I can here.

As we progress through this book and look at adult outcomes for autistic women, we will see that intelligence does not necessarily lead to a conventionally successful outcome. Many autistic women have to find their own rocky path to their own version of success, which may come later and in a different form to anything anyone could have predicted from that bright, quiet, helpful bookworm of a girl.

On the whole, the girls and autistic women who participated in the research for this book – particularly those diagnosed in adulthood – had a rotten time in their school years due to a lack of early diagnosis, support and any understanding of their perception of the school experience. This knowledge is useful in enabling us to identify how they felt and what went wrong for them, and to put measures in place to prevent other autistic girls from having the same experiences. This is a hope shared by one autistic mother for her daughter:

> It was a long road to get my daughter recognized as being on the spectrum. Once support is in place, the difference is remarkable; I am almost envious and wish that I had had this understanding. It is my mission that she will not end up like me. Her home will be her haven, she will find love, understanding and support from her parents, and I will insist that her school does the same. All of her desires and interests are supported; I cannot bear the thought of her feeling frustrated like I did. I look back and wonder what I could have been, had my interests been indulged.

Starting school

It is sometimes not until a child begins some form of formal education that their autistic profile starts to become apparent. All children have their own quirks and preferences, which are met and managed within the home and the family – especially given the genetic likelihood that parents and other family members may also be autistic – and it may not be until the child is required to tolerate a large number of other children plus a few strangers for several hours a day that problems arise. She may have been an active helper to her parents at home, polite and talkative to visitors, relaxed and outgoing with her family and happy organizing her toys and collections – a child who showed no signs of visible stress, because there probably wasn't any. When asked about their experiences of their children starting pre-school, parents of autistic girls report:

> Starting school was awful. Up until this time she was a happy, lovely little girl. The anxiety she feels is very upsetting. To be honest, I think she has resigned herself to school. I will consider home school when she is older if she finds it too difficult; the damage it could cause her is something I know only too well.

> [...] Dreadful. It was then that we started to really see the differences.

Some children have no concept of why they are going to this new place. It may seem obvious to us that this is simply 'the way things are' after a certain age, but this assumption cannot be made for an autistic child. We may assume that the socializing aspect of play settings is beneficial to the child. This is an almost universally held belief, particularly in the case of girls. The autistic child may disagree. It may be that for some autistic children there really is no point or functional benefit in them attending a group play setting and that the distress caused outweighs any possible benefit gained. This notion is difficult for many parents to acknowledge as they believe that being alone cannot be good for the child; but for many children and autistic adults, being alone is the best thing of all.

> I was distraught and in tears and didn't want to go. I didn't see the point. I would regularly vomit in the car on the way to pre-school.

> I would watch her through the window when I came to collect her. She was always alone sitting quietly engrossed in whatever she was doing whilst the other children ran and shouted together around her. (Parent)

> When I returned to collect her, the staff were wearing ear defenders. I thought it was some kind of construction game with the children, but it turned out that she had been screaming for the past two hours and they couldn't cope. I had not had any mobile signal and had not heard their desperate attempts to reach me to come and get her. (Parent)

Capacity can become stretched for the first time in the child's life, and very different behaviours may be observed. For the child herself, the world has suddenly changed beyond all recognition and has potentially become very frightening; she has had to leave her home (her sanctuary), and in its place there is this cacophonous, labyrinthine, stranger-filled abyss. In the responses to my questions, there was a marked difference between those who were diagnosed in adulthood, who had to navigate school without a label or any adjustments, and those who were diagnosed in childhood and received support (although this may have been hard fought for by their parents and initially traumatic for the child).

> The transition to pre-school was very difficult. She became upset and didn't want to go in [...] The manager asked me to stay every day for three weeks, and then I gradually stayed for less and less time. [The manager] said that she had never had a child who reacted like this for such a long time. The transition to primary school was much better. We knew that she probably was autistic at this stage, and a comprehensive transition plan was put into place. She settled in quickly and enjoyed it. (Parent)

Eileen Riley-Hall (2012) advises parents to take a photograph of their daughter to any meeting to discuss her education in order to remind everyone present that she 'is a person, not just a programme to be created in a cost-effective manner' (p.49).

The adult-diagnosed women's recollections are, in the vast majority of cases, negative and painful to read: 'dreadful', 'awful', 'horrific' and 'distraught' are the words they use. For parents of children who have managed to get support in place, the story is remarkably different and positive but sadly rare. Comparing these experiences lends huge hope and support to the idea that knowledge and a change in attitude can make a real difference for the daily experience of the autistic child. The tales of late-diagnosed women give insight into a world that we should not be subjecting an autistic child to in the present day.

> I remember early on [...] crying and hiding behind a door when we walked from one classroom to a new classroom and I was unaware of what was going to happen.

> My mum says I hated nursery. She never managed to leave me there for a full day as the teachers often had to call her because I was crying so much.

> [...] Horrific, traumatic experience, which sadly never improved.

> The school environment was stressful and hectic and full of people who seemed to hate me for no reason.

Many of the comments and experiences here could apply to all genders, but some are more indicative of the female profile and of others' expectations of girls' behaviour and social abilities, which these girls may not be able (or aspire) to match up to. It is difficult to convey just how deep-seated and a core part of society these gender expectations are, and how hard it is to consciously recognize these girls and be willing to view them as different but equally acceptable just as they are.

There are many books on educating children on the autism spectrum, with tips, tools and techniques that go into great depth.

I will touch on a few here, but my main purpose is to illustrate the female experience in a school setting. The intention is not to frighten professionals or parents of young autistic girls into seeing the horrors that lie ahead; rather, it is to prevent these experiences happening to future generations of girls. The headings below are not consistent across each educational setting as different aspects cause different levels of difficulty at different stages. I would advise that reading through all settings might be worthwhile to get a picture of potential issues in education as a whole rather than just isolating one age group. Any child or adult with whom you are working either will have already experienced much of what is discussed through these sections, or has yet to do so as they move forward through the education system. Either way, a holistic consideration of the impact of their past and potential future should enable any professional to better consider appropriate educational measures to be put in place.

Early Years – pre-school, nursery and playgroup

Structure

Early Years settings can be quite fluid and flexible in their schedules, which may cause additional difficulties for the autistic child who does not know what is going to happen unless explicitly told. Some children become distressed at their parent leaving them at playgroup or school because no one informed them that the parent would return. Without the benefit of imagination, the child may assume that she will never see her parent again, which makes the level of distress understandable in that context.

Some level of predictability and timetabling might help an autistic child to cope with knowing what to expect each day and how and when it will start and end. Explicit and visual reassurance can support the child in managing her own anxious feelings.

> At playgroup, she seemed to find unstructured play unsettling. Was often telling the adults that they were wrong, e.g. spelling or simple facts (usually correctly!). Was seen as aloof and a bit posh!

A pictorial schedule of the day pinned to the wall might provide evidence of certainty, and the child can be encouraged to learn where to find the information she needs on it. This may also give the child the chance to look forward to certain activities and encourage her to attend – particularly if these can be tailored to meet the child's interests. Being told that tomorrow she will be able to look at pictures of cats and draw cats – if cats are her 'thing' – may help a reluctant child to feel motivated to attend. In terms of other motivators, it may be that social ones don't work. As we shall see below, other children were often the cause of difficulty and apprehension about attending school or nursery. Attempting to persuade an autistic girl to go to playgroup in order to 'play with her friends' might remind her of the horror of sharing toys and reduce her to tears and panic. For many autistic children, free playtime is the hardest time of all to manage. Identifying the motivators that are meaningful to her – interests, favourite carer, specific toys, biscuits at breaktime and chocolate on the journey home if she makes it through the day – is most likely to achieve success.

Teaching and support staff

Early Years settings are often partly staffed by volunteers, who may have limited or no knowledge or experience of ASD – particularly as it is often not diagnosed in this age group unless there are significant verbal or global developmental indicators. In contrast, they may have plenty of knowledge about how they expect a neurotypical child of this age to behave. These general expectations of what is typical can put pressure on the child to conform in ways that are unmanageably difficult for them, but with nobody around them knowing why they become so distressed. A requirement to sit on an itchy carpet, touch wet sand or hold hands with another child may make the setting unbearable for an autistic child.

> They [staff] insisted on tying my hair up, and I found this very painful. Until recently when I read about autistic people having scalp sensitivity, I blamed them for being horrid and pulling my hair so painfully.

Training and awareness for staff working in these settings are crucial in ensuring early positive experiences for young autistic girls, even if the ASD is only suspected by the parent at this stage. Diagnosis is unlikely to have taken place for many of these girls at this age, but early signs of difference should be accommodated, regardless of official recognition. It may be possible to make only limited adjustments to the environment due to factors outside the Early Years organizer's control, but small measures can make a huge difference: a quiet space being made available with headphones, being permitted to hold a teacher's belt rather than her hand, wearing rubber gloves while playing in the sand pit, a beanbag and a favourite toy are strategies that might provide a small respite and reduce anxiety for a child who is feeling overwhelmed or overloaded.

Physical environment

This is a young girl's first experience of spending significant time with people other than her family and in an unfamiliar environment. In the UK, these Early Years experiences may sometimes take place in a building that is not built as a place of learning and which is used for many functions throughout the day – a church hall, Scout hut or leisure centre, for example. The rooms are often large, old and have strange acoustics. Furniture and equipment have to be set out and packed away at the start and end of each session, and that can mean that materials and space may be limited and not very adaptable. The impact of these factors on an autistic child may be that they experience stress around the sensory environment in terms of noise and acoustics, but also in terms of a lack of consistency about the layout of the space. I have worked with children (and adults) who cannot tolerate furniture being moved in a classroom without their presence; for them it is like entering an entirely different place and requires them to completely reconfigure their understanding of where they are every time they enter the room. Something as simple as this could result in anxiety and so-called 'challenging behaviour' due to total disorientation and panic.

School

The transition from an Early Years setting into school can be quite a shock for an autistic child. A uniform with all its required sensory tolerance may be insisted upon, the length of the school day may increase two-fold and the afternoon nap is a thing of the past. Although some autistic children embrace the clear rules, structure and boundaries that school imposes, since these things provide routine and hence a sense of safety and relief, others find the number of people and the length of the school day extremely difficult to manage. Good preparation for this, prior to the child starting school, is essential to ensure that the child understands what school involves and has some idea of the environment that she will be spending her days in. Teachers reported that autistic males externalize their social problems more readily than females and therefore are more likely to be identified as needing support in the classroom (Mandy *et al.*, 2012).

> She finds school emotionally draining [...] she would often 'explode' the minute she left the school gate and I learned that it was best not to speak to her at all while we walked home because any conversation would lead to meltdown. (Parent)

It is necessary to remember that the autistic girl may not appear to have any difficulties due to her ability to camouflage and compensate; she may be the ideal child, helpful and polite. This may be the case at first, but as she gets older and additional demands are made of her, both socially and educationally, the mask may start to slip. It has been shown that increased demands in both areas contribute to increased anxiety in autistic girls (Stewart, 2012). And, as we have seen, when the mask slips, something that looks like mental health issues can be revealed; however, careful observation may lead to the conclusion that changes in a girl's behaviour are simply the result of an inability to maintain the neurotypical persona that she has learned to create. An important thing to note, and that has been seen in this research and elsewhere (e.g. Stewart, 2012), is that autistic girls want to do well, comply and not get into trouble. As professionals, if we always keep in mind that when a girl is doing something that on the face of it appears rude, diffident or downright obstructive, she is, in fact, trying her hardest to do the right thing, regardless of how it might appear, and we can support her by understanding what she is trying to say or do and teach her a new way of doing it in the future.

Learning and teaching style

Many of the women and girls who participated in this book were precocious early talkers, often with extensive vocabularies. This does not mean that learning came/comes easily to them, on account of the neurotypical system they were/are expected to adhere to. We must not forget that, even in a learning environment, social requirements are always present, which means that our autistic girl has to work doubly hard to make sense of both the social and the academic elements.

> I had little interest in other children and would much rather have been left alone with books to study by myself or just have one-to-one lessons. Being around the other children was a huge impediment to my learning, well-being and mental health.

> Due to my constant daydreaming and struggles following spoken instructions, I had a lot of trouble with learning.

> I was pretty good academically; my biggest difficulty was probably with my own arrogance, and I felt I was superior to not only the other kids but to the teacher.

We know that autistic individuals find life easier if there is some structure and predictability about what's coming next. It means that anxiety is reduced, and therefore the capacity and ability for learning are increased. School is often full of rituals, routines and structures. Unfortunately, many of these make little sense as they may have a social or compliance basis rather than a logical one. They may also be imposed without any contextual explanation to enable the child to learn why these social behaviours are beneficial and/or necessary. Being reprimanded for not doing something that you didn't know you had to do and why you had to do it – and hence are unlikely to understand the context of when to do it next time – causes anxiety. Knowing that you will undoubtedly get something 'wrong', but are not sure what or when, is perhaps why autistic children can develop school phobia.

It is thought that autistic girls are more likely to suffer in silence (Wagner, 2006) and that their 'shy' profile means their learning difficulties go unnoticed. These girls may just be seen as poorly performing students. The desire to fit in and not be seen as stupid by their peers may explain a reluctance to raise their hands to answer a question or to stand out in any way.

> If teachers ask if she is okay, [she] will just say yes even if [she] is not okay; [she] won't ask for help at school. (Parent)

> She is a perfectionist [...] she would not put up her hand or answer a question for many years in case she was wrong [...] She generally sits at the back saying very little but still manages to produce excellent work. (Parent)

> She won't speak to a teacher because she 'doesn't want to bother them' and 'might get shouted at'. This is a problem because she will never ask if she doesn't understand. (Parent)

Subjects

Among those women questioned, art and English topped the list of favourite subjects at school. These are not the typically expected 'male' ASD topics (usually involving maths and IT), which may add to the difficulty in considering an ASD diagnosis for a literary and creative girl. Many were voracious readers and most happy when engrossed in a book during the school day. They also enjoyed drawing and colouring – perceived as typical female pursuits. Gathering factual (or fictional) information in a solo world appears to be more enjoyable than gathering social information in the real world for these girls, and their knowledge of chosen subjects can be extensive. My personal experience was of being constantly described as 'lazy' by teachers for never achieving an 'A' grade despite being a gifted-level student with precocious early speech. I have always said that I knew the answer, but I didn't know the question. It was other people's language I had trouble with, not my own. Language processing (verbal and written) made much of learning inaccessible, but I was fortunate to be able to scrape through using intellect and logic, which has its limitations. This remains the same in my adult life.

Autistic girls, like their male peers, can show unusual, uneven learning profiles, where instead of having a fairly consistent profile of ability, they exhibit extreme subject-area peaks and troughs. The causes of this can be a combination of:

- the cognitive profile of autism itself
- the nature of the subject being taught
- the individual's natural processing style and ability
- the teaching style
- the level of interest and motivation that the student has in the topic.

All or some of these elements can combine to create a greater or lesser ability in certain subjects. If the subject content is inaccessible, due to either its nature or the way in which it is taught, an autistic student is more likely to switch off and feel incapable of engaging. The logical nature of autistic people leads some to conclude that if they know they are going to fail at something, why bother to even try?

> I saw little point in doing any subject I wasn't good at as it seemed a waste of time and just an exercise in futility and self-humiliation.

> She has lost her way with most subjects and doesn't get on with

> how the subjects are taught. She is very bright and able but now finds it hard to understand what the teachers are trying to communicate. Since she realized that nothing actually happens when she doesn't do the work, she stopped properly trying.

Something as simple as considering a different teaching approach or explaining a broader contextual reason for the purpose of the topic can bring about a change in attitude and performance in certain subjects. Sadly, it appears to be the norm that support in school has to be hard fought for by parents, and if the child is struggling for too long, it may be difficult to bring her back to a place where she can continue to learn.

> A support plan was implemented recently...[my] daughter was able to sit with a good friend in class and teachers have been instructed on how to support her learning, but it is too little too late. After pressure from me, her timetable has been reduced, but her anxiety is such that she is barely engaging. (Parent)

Teaching staff

Research has shown that teachers are less likely to notice and/or report difficulties with adapting in autistic girls than boys (Mandy *et al.*, 2012), perhaps due to the invisible presentation in girls and the perception of ASD as a male condition. Autistic girls have been found to exhibit less restricted, stereotyped behaviours, which are a known visible sign of potential autism. It may well be that if a teacher does not notice any such behaviour, they may not be open to the possibility of autism being present. Teachers rarely have sufficient knowledge of autism, even less so its presentation in girls (Wagner, 2006). Constant misunderstandings from teachers were a common theme in the responses of my participants and have also been identified as a concern elsewhere. Dr Catriona Stewart OBE states that:

> As they worked to establish a system of rules that allowed them to function (i.e. systems of behaviour relating to logic,

> sustainability, cause and effect, predictable outcomes, fairness), the girls were expected to function in a world of people whose behaviour did not adhere to them. (2012, p.42)

These misunderstandings were also referred to by others:

> I did well in school but did not speak a lot and ended up in detention for really [trivial] things like [refusing to talk].

> Before we had the diagnosis our life was hell...we knew that there were problems but we didn't have a diagnosis and that was really hard work with the teachers. We changed her schools because they just seemed to think that she was a bad kid... We were so isolated from the whole community because people just looked at us as bad people and looked at her as a bad child. (Parent) (Cridland *et al.*, 2014, p.1265)

> She tells me how she was sent to the Principal's office because she had kicked someone under the table. She says she didn't know why she was there or what she had done – she was just swinging her legs. (Parent)

> We were playing a game where everyone stands in a line with their feet apart, and the person at the front rolls a ball through everyone's legs to be caught by the last person in the line, who runs to the front [...] The teacher pulled me out of the line and shook me in front of everyone, and I never did understand what for.

Teachers are predominantly female, and perhaps – given their people-focused, flexible, communication-based career choice – may be quite different in personality from their young, female autistic charges. When one considers the difficulties that these girls can have with their female peers, it shouldn't surprise us that they have similar problems with the grown-up versions of those peers, who may become teachers! It is also important to remember that relationships are reciprocal, so it is not simply the case that the autistic girl doesn't understand and relate well to her more intuitively communicative teacher; it is equally the case that the teacher may not feel that she has 'connected' with this unusual (especially so for a 'girl') child. The standard reciprocal 'positive strokes' may not be there, and the teacher may be confused by their feelings about this girl. Autistic children may also be highly knowledgeable in certain subjects and, not perceiving the invisible social rules of hierarchy, may quite confidently correct or interject when a teacher is speaking. This can be perceived as a deliberate attempt at insult by a teacher, whereas the girl is simply presenting empirical facts and has no agenda to cause emotional harm or any understanding that she may be doing so. This unintentional breaking of 'covert social conventions' can mean that these girls are labelled as 'intentionally disruptive' by teachers, which can lead to them feeling that they can never fit in socially, however hard they try (Tierney *et al.*, 2016).

> I was always pointing out everyone's mistakes, including any words that teachers spelled wrong on the whiteboard... In high school, noticing errors made me unpopular. Later, rising through the ranks of a marketing and web development company, it became my job to ensure that everyone else's work was technically correct. (Kotowicz, 2022, p.17)

As professionals, it is essential that people self-reflect and separate their – often strong – personal feelings towards a person from their professional duty to do the right thing for that individual. I am not aware that teacher-training programmes include this type of practice, but it is my belief that they should. It may be that the teacher is not even aware of why this child upsets them so much as it can occur on a subconscious level. People who are very emotionally intuitive can sometimes take the behaviour of this type of girl personally and assume that she is deliberately trying to make life difficult. The insights from autistic girls and women reveal that this is seldom, if ever, the case. Mostly, they are desperate to get it right and gain approval and acceptance, but despite their best efforts, they often appear to do the one thing that causes a teacher to react very badly to them at times.

> They [teachers] didn't like me, thought I was lazy, and often accused me [of] being an attention-seeker, when all I really did was actually avoid everyone.

> Some [teachers] felt her rude/insolent when she showed high levels of knowledge and intelligence. (Parent)

> They [teachers] seemed to think I was choosing to be different and to have social difficulties [...] One teacher bullied me terribly and used to reprimand me for not giving him eye contact.

It is worth noting that there is often an expectation that girls will be more skilled than boys at social niceties and so may be judged differently – and sometimes more harshly – when they fail to behave in a 'nice' way on occasions where their intentions may have been misinterpreted. The following is a good example of this:

> I wanted to surprise my friend by taking her outside and getting her to feel the rain in her face. She was still in the classroom, so I covered her eyes and took her out of the class, walking blindly, while telling her it was a surprise. As we walked down onto the patio she tripped, fell on a muddy patch, and her uniform got dirty. A teacher noticed and came over. She called me a 'nasty, ugly girl'. I was not given the chance to explain, nor had I the verbal skills to interrupt and explain what I had intended to do. I had had no malicious intent whatsoever.

Social interaction

For many autistic children, breaktime is the most difficult part of the school day. The structure of the lesson is gone, and the entire population of the school is released into the playground, our girl included. Suddenly, social abilities reign supreme, and an understanding of the complexities of relationships, negotiation and rules of play is required. It would be fair to say that our autistic girl may well return to the classroom after a 'break' more exhausted than she was when she left it. This is an extremely important point and one that must be considered in reflecting on behaviour, performance and general well-being at school.

> [The playground] was noisy, unorganized chaos. I went home for lunches and avoided busy [areas] at playtime.

> I wanted to stay in and read a book but was not allowed. I spent most playtimes alone.

> I would stand by the punishment wall (a place where kids were sent to stand if they had done bad things) every playtime of every day, and do nothing but stand there during that time.

> Playtime remains difficult for my daughter. We asked the school to give her more supervision, [and] access to a quiet area indoors: a place for her to eat her lunch outside the dining hall at times of high anxiety as these things are very hard for her. (Parent)

As girls get older, their friendships change, and they move away from toy-based, pretence games to more sophisticated people- and personality-based relationships. Girls talk about other girls (and boys); their relationships are subtle and nuanced and allegiances are forever changing. Autistic girls struggle increasingly with age to, first, understand why this change has occurred – they were quite happy as things were – and, second, to be able to continue to hold their own in this new social arena (Riley-Hall, 2012). Girls can feel a lack of safety in being surrounded by 'feeling at the mercy of more powerful others, broadly conceptualized as those who understood the social rules' (Tierney *et al.*, 2016, p.76), some even going so far as to describe the school experience as 'predatory' and expressing a feeling of being 'ungirly' in comparison to their female peers.

> It feels like in my classroom that I am surrounded by lions... I feel like a mouse and everyone else is a giant cat or something. (Tierney *et al.*, 2016, p.76)

School breaktime is the primary location for this new terror – and it happens three times a day. This is supposed to be the part of the day that is 'fun'! For parents, the expectation may be that seeing friends after school is a natural thing for their child to want to do. The parent of one girl explains beautifully the perspective of her daughter with regard to socializing after school:

> We rarely had playdates in the first couple of years because she said, 'I've been at school with people all day – why would I want to see them again now?' (Parent)

The main problem for young autistic women at school during the teenage years is their social relationships and ability to be around other people for extended periods of time. The challenges of earlier childhood school remain but are exacerbated by an increased awareness of the difference between them and their peers. Spending time surrounded by teenagers at school is a constant reminder of these feelings of difference, and it is unavoidable.

> I was totally lost as a teen at school, I had no idea how to pull off fitting in and didn't want to be like the others. I wanted school to be about learning exciting, interesting stuff and then the subject matter being what everyone talked about, but alas that wasn't the case. School seemed to be one big social experience, and the learning and subject matter were irrelevant to most people.

> When things were fine the autism helped my education – memory, numerical skill, etc. But when things went wrong people were quick to judge things as 'hormonal/emotional problems'

> or 'attention seeking' rather than listen to me try to explain the actual issues.

> Sharing space was a problem. I didn't care to be around others much and during the teenage years – at school, home and work – I was trapped with people, which was horrendous for me. I used to spend ages in the bathroom with the door locked as it was the only place I could be alone with my thoughts.

Physical environment

> For a lot of school, we sat alone at desks, not in groups. This was perfect for me.

For many young autistic women, the physical environment of mainstream school is extremely stressful (Stewart, 2012), and this gets worse as they grow older. School dining halls are notoriously overwhelming for autistic children, mainly because of the noise (cutlery, scraping chairs, banging plates, incessant chatter) but also because of the smell, visual overload and social elements (where shall I sit?). This stress can be exacerbated when there is the requirement to navigate the complex female social world of working out allegiances and non-verbal signals. One girl did not eat at lunchtime because the dining area was intolerable for her (Stewart, 2012) leading to potential health issues. Corridors can cause distress when having to move from one classroom to another (Tierney *et al.*, 2016) due to increased sensory stimulation and sensitivity.

Further education

College

> I had convinced myself that my high IQ and high academic achievement record meant I was strong enough to handle whatever came my way [...] I was hit hard when I had to realize smarts

> were not enough to make it in this world. I was turned upside down when I had to admit I could not find anyone who saw things like I did. (Liane Holliday Willey, 2014, p.63)

Liane writes of how she had an accepting group of friends at school and how she expected to find the same at college, but instead found herself floundering in a bigger, unknown environment. While being bullied often decreases as people get older, it can be replaced with invisibility, which feels like rejection, regardless of intent. College means starting over again, with the need to initiate new relationships, but these are more adult, and more socially nuanced, than the last time that this had to be done at the start of school.

Some women in my survey found that college was easier than school as there is more freedom of movement, there are fewer classes per day and you are able to choose to study subjects that you excel at and enjoy. The more mature treatment of students at college suits some autistic individuals – those who like control and autonomy and simply to be left alone. A few found kindred spirits in their tutors, who offered knowledge and an escape.

> I found it much easier to deal with college. When you are at school you cannot be alone at lunch/breaktimes, but at college it's seen as quite acceptable to go to the library, or study or sit quietly and read a book.

> I spent a considerable amount of time chatting to one of my lecturers, who was, on reflection, obviously on the [autism] spectrum [...] If it wasn't for him, I don't think I would have achieved my A-levels. His office was like a sanctuary for me.

University

The challenges of university for autistic women are largely similar to those of all genders of autistic people, and other writing focuses on these aspects in greater detail. For women, the specific difficulties remain the same as for other areas of life: social interaction with female peers, mental health problems as a result of difficulties coping with what is required of them and lack of diagnosis, and, therefore, lack of understanding or support of any kind. The key to a successful experience of university appears for many young women to be linked to social integration and acceptance. They may have the academic abilities to undertake the work, but the isolation and implicit rejection can make the difference between successful completion and dropping out. Personal relationship issues are discussed elsewhere but might also be a contributory factor during this time.

> When I went to university, I failed my first year. The other students were girly girls; I just did not fit in. I felt very lonely and missed tons of lectures and deadlines. They failed me but allowed me to re-sit the year [...] Thankfully, I got together with a group of students.

> We were a bunch of misfits [...] We had a great time – those three years were brilliant. I felt completely accepted in my circle of friends and successfully completed my degree, with a few deadline extensions!

> I'm doing a distance learning course, so I don't really have to interact much with people. The occasional presentation or Skype discussion I can cope with, although I'm very self-conscious about these and find them stressful.

> My autism wasn't diagnosed until after university. I feel that had I been a male child, it would have been picked up sooner [...] At university, I was mentally ill, and I struggled to cope socially too as I don't drink and I don't go to clubs or pubs. I didn't speak to anyone other than my tutors for the first year and nearly left on several occasions. When I tried to interact with people or be open about my difficulties and distress, people just became exasperated and bored with me, like I was a nuisance rather than someone desperate for support.

Educational support

> It's also hard because she is different from the students in mainstream but being a girl makes her different from the kids in the Autism Unit too, she doesn't fit in anywhere. (Parent) (Cridland *et al.*, 2014, p.1265)

Although every girl and young autistic woman will need an individualized support plan to meet her needs, there are a number of general approaches that teachers can adopt that will certainly aid the child's process of transition and settling into a new educational setting:

- Put the support in place before she starts at your school.
- Meet her before she starts, show her around – let her know where she will be and what's required. Find her a pal to help her find her way into the social side of things.
- Use visuals, schedules and other concrete information to help her settle in and make sense of what will happen and when.
- Autistic girls generally want to do well, comply and stay out of trouble. If this is not happening, the chances are she has a gap in her understanding of what's required. Remember this before reacting.
- Do not take what she says or does personally. She is not meaning to annoy you. (If she is unable to predict the thoughts and feelings of others, she won't have a clue how to wind you up.)
- Consider your rules. Are you and others adhering to them? She will be – sometimes in a very literal and black-and-white way. The rules that she has been given may be all she has to navigate the world. The fact that others don't appear to have to stick to them will distress and confuse her greatly.

- Staff need training in autism and specifically how it manifests in girls.
- Don't assume that because she's smart (or average) she will be fine. She won't. All the qualifications in the world don't mean a thing if you can't hold a conversation without masking or anxiety.
- Teach the non-academic skills – even if you have a doctorate, you still need to be able to answer a phone or make the tea. She may not be able to do either of these things.
- Consider language-processing limitations – just because she is highly articulate (her words) doesn't mean that she can comprehend what you require (your words). One does not equal the other – often it is completely the opposite. She is literal and eloquent purely because it's the one and only way that she understands the concept.
- Pre-teach the content of lessons. Give her the heads-up on the topic area in advance and let her go and research it on her own. In this way, she will have had time to process the information, reducing surprises and increasing her ability to participate in the lessons. Do this with all your students.
- Ensure that she understands the requirements of assignments. Provide her with parameters and guidelines on length, content, timescale and priority so that she doesn't spend too long striving for perfection when it's not necessary.
- Keep an eye on her. She may not ask for help. Asking for help may equate to weakness or failure. She may not know that she needs help or know that help is available.
- Bring her interests into the curriculum. You will see her true ability and potential when you have her full engagement with a topic. Be creative – many interests can be encompassed in many subjects:
  - counting Pokémon

  - English language essays based on cats
  - horse care in the 19th century.

- If teamwork is necessary, give her a role that she can succeed in. Don't let her have to try to negotiate with others (social skills) to find her place. Do this with all the students if you don't want to single her out. Let them all be successful in areas where their strengths lie. She is likely to excel in planning, research and possibly writing up results.
- Reduce homework assignments. She is exhausted.

Chapter 11

EMPLOYMENT

> *I would get into trouble because I wasn't socializing enough. I was so efficient that I could finish my work by 11 a.m., but then I'd have to sit there until 5 just talking to people and pretending to be productive.*
>
> Autistic woman

It is widely believed that autistic individuals have difficulties in both obtaining and retaining employment for a number of reasons, most of which relate to them being autistic in workplaces where this is misunderstood or not accepted for the great benefit that it could bring. There are several books on this topic, including one I wrote (Hendrickx, 2009). For this book, I found a bunch of autistic people who had been successful in their very various working lives and tried to find the patterns that may have led to their success. At the time, this seemed rather ground-breaking, but with the greater knowledge that many autistic people have of themselves and their needs/skills, it all seems rather obvious. I 'discovered' that autistic people like to do things that really interest them in environments that don't make them feel ill and with people who largely leave them alone. In most cases, the autistic people I spoke to had not known that they were autistic when they began their working lives, and by chance, luck, trial and error they had ended up in workplaces that were perfect for them. Obviously, there is more to the book than that (buy it, buy it, my poorly planned retirement depends on it!), but in essence autistic people like autistic jobs. Now that we have established this possibly glaring obvious fact, it should come as no surprise not only that are these types of jobs quite hard to find, but also that autistic women often 1) don't know that they are autistic, 2) are too busy trying to do the same jobs that everyone else does to ever consider whether it is making them ill, and if it is making them ill, 3) are too busy to consider that this is in any way unusual because every job they've ever had has made them feel ill in one way or another.

> I had mental health breakdowns, not understood to be autistic burnouts, in every job I've ever had, which is the main reason I left each employment. I assumed I couldn't cope with the job, so I had to leave. No one offered any support; I didn't know why I was struggling to ask for support, so I just continued in a vicious circle throughout my 'career'.

> I get physical feelings of anxiety. I have learned to hold it in when in the workplace, although not always successfully, and have spent many a lunch hour hiding in the work toilets hyper-ventilating and sobbing uncontrollably. I used to feel pathetic when this happened; I now realize since diagnosis how incredibly brave I was, actually pulling myself together and going back to work for the afternoon, before collapsing through my front door when I got home, feeling such distress and anxiety.

Sixty per cent of autistic women reported that the social aspects of work were one of the worst things about their experience of employment. They describe that simple communication and social interaction with colleagues can feel draining and overwhelming (Baldwin and Costley, 2016). Twenty-three per cent of the women in this study reported bullying to be a problem for them with people making jokes and calling them 'mad/weird/different'.

> I certainly didn't have any female friends at work, was often left out of social invitations and mocked for not being girly enough. I definitely got on better with male colleagues, which often led

> to my enjoyment of their company being misunderstood and becoming awkward with relationships either started and ended, or I declined their advances.

As someone who has had more than 40 jobs, I can relate to these challenges. My reasons for leaving each one, often with no other form of income to take its place despite at times being on my own with children to support, I can see were all related to me being autistic. I walked out of jobs over matters of principle where I was unable to tolerate the injustice I saw, either towards me or others. I walked out because I couldn't cope with banter, teasing and my inability to socialize with my colleagues in the way that was expected. I refused to go to a Christmas party and was threatened with being fired, my work was stolen and used by a colleague without credit given to me, and I was bullied and made fun of and told that I couldn't take a joke. I couldn't follow rules that made no sense; I had no concept of hierarchy and would tell my bosses how to run their companies because it was so obvious to me that they were doing it wrong. I also once bought my CEO a Mr. Potato Head for a secret Santa (he was bald). He knew it was me.

> I have 100 per cent conversion rate from interview to being offered the job, probably due to learning how to behave / what to say in an interview, but within six months of each job, my mask would begin to slip, my absences would get more frequent and I would eventually leave before I was sacked.

Steph Jones, an autistic therapist who also set up the Autism Professionals Network, also sees clients with regard to their experiences of autistic burnout in the workplace. She says that it is often not the job tasks themselves that are causing the problem, but the low-level interactions required, the environment and the need to switch tasks repeatedly. Lunch breaks for autistic women may be necessary for recharging in order to face the afternoon, whereas female peers may judge her for being aloof or rude for not wishing to share the social time together and build the rapport expected to be a 'team player'. Without this respite, there may be no chance to recover from the morning before doing it all over again in the afternoon. Several women describe how they would cry in the toilets from the effort of getting through the day with their mask intact.

> I could never hold an office job for long. I either got fired or I quit. I thought the problem was me; that I hadn't found the right thing. I could be great and charming for an hour, maybe two, then I would power down like a robot and be rude to customers. I would become bone-deep exhausted and so irritated I couldn't even lift my mouth to smile. My boss said 'smile or leave', so I left. This kind of interaction happened over and over again. I could do great work until 11 a.m. and then I'd be in the bathroom having a panic attack and meditating to calm myself down. I know now that eight hours around people is just not an option for me any more. (Schembari, 2023)

> I think that I've managed to struggle by in employment for so long because I became so good at faking it. In fact, over the past few years this has caused me a lot of anguish because it had got to the stage where even I no longer knew who was behind the mask, and I began to fear I was going mad because I just didn't seem to know who I was any more.

One Australian study found that 55 per cent of autistic women were employed in positions where their qualifications exceeded that of the job role (the overall figure for all Australian women is 24%) (Baldwin and Costley, 2016). In the same study, 86 per cent of autistic women expressed a preference for working part time for various reasons including a feeling that working full time was unmanageable for them. A study of diagnosticians assessing autistic women also noted that they had often failed to achieve expected levels of professional or personal success (Cumin *et al.*, 2022). Other women found that working at all was simply not possible.

> I haven't felt able to work for over ten years, and I now know that this is not because I am lazy, but because I find juggling the whole work experience with life too much to process and deal with.

> I work below my ability and qualifications to reduce the amount of stress I am under, and I can only work part time.

> I find the office politics a bit of a minefield, as well as the social graces and 'brown nosing' to get on rather than being judged on capabilities. I have tended to do menial jobs and was self-employed for 16 years.

> I never stayed in a company/role long enough to be progressed or promoted, so I effectively moved companies at the same level the whole time I've been employed.

> My lack of ability to bullshit or big myself up and my poor interview skills hold me back. I am very able but do find that I think differently to others, which can lead to misunderstandings.

> Historically I've struggled to stay in jobs very long. The main issue is that things have gone wrong as I've not understood the dynamics and got myself into difficult situations that were uncomfortable or been unclear as to what was required of me, and then not met expectations / people got upset as I did what I thought they wanted.

Work has the potential to be one of the single greatest challenges for autistic women due to the long-term nature of the social relationships that you are required to develop whether you want them or not, the physical environment that you must endure on a daily basis and the infinite potential for unexpected situations and change. The sheer effort of having to be somewhere other than home, often surrounded by people you didn't choose, for most of your waking hours is certainly a trigger for autistic burnout, despite most of the population coping with this without significant harm. Social and networking expectations can prove difficult for some women in the workplace. Much like elsewhere in the world, there are hidden agendas, social boundaries and hierarchies to be understood and adhered to.

> I never understood management hierarchy, often hearing 'you can't say that to them', but not understanding why, which resulted in not being able to communicate with certain people for fear of saying the wrong thing.

> I struggled to work in a team as other people mostly did a pretty poor job compared to my ability/expectation, so I would get frustrated and either lash out verbally, refuse to do the work or take control so people did things my way.

> I ducked out of the mainstream accounting career after a few years as I couldn't understand the dynamics of working in practice. There were always lots of games being played, and I never understood what they were, let alone the rules.

> In the self-employed world I struggle with the networking aspect (which is important to find new clients) and social media as I don't understand the rules. NTs [neurotypicals] say be honest and be vulnerable to be authentic, but I'm pretty sure they don't mean it – it seems like curated authenticity.

> I'm usually seen as being the one who is great with customers. Which is a pain because I find customer-facing work exhausting. I like things to work well, and I like people to feel welcomed and respected. But I'd much rather do that in the background than performing out front.

One of the difficulties mentioned by the women I questioned related to information processing and multi-tasking. It is presumed that women can manage multiple instructions and conversations and take on board new information quickly and flexibly. This is not always the case for autistic women, who may be very adept at structured, linear tasks and information but take longer and require more detail for abstract information (such as directions and procedures).

> I think that people misunderstanding me has made major, negative impacts; employers have always misunderstood me and not believed me when I've told them what I can and can't do. I can work alone, I can work in teams and I can lead teams; and I can do any of those roles while being efficient, positive and respectful. However, if people don't explain things properly, won't provide relevant context or written instructions, refuse to follow agreed systems, expect me to multi-task or won't support sensory accommodations, things fall apart quickly.

> I often felt as though almost every member of staff [was] giving me instructions, and often one would be telling me to do the opposite of the other. I often felt as though I was on the receiving end of many people who saw me as their opportunity to be in control [...] I was slower than other members of staff at understanding things and therefore more at the mercy of every person in a workplace who dreamed of being a boss.

> I am new to office life, and I feel with most things it starts off well but then you are expected to master everything. I am still getting lost in the building and asking questions about things others are clear on.

> I often have a meltdown every year when it comes to organizing my financial information to send to my accountant. I get rather muddled when it comes to bureaucracy and what needs to be done or remembered... New rules and regulations...have had quite an impact on my neurodivergent brain, creating another layer of processing and anxiety.

Autistic women often have a strong sense of fairness and justice and a desire to abide by the stipulated rules. This may bring them into conflict with colleagues who may not be doing the same. This can cause enormous stress, which may make the woman leave the employment or result in her displaying her blunt, outspoken side. An autistic woman may not be able to 'keep quiet' if she feels that a situation is plain wrong. Office politics and 'sucking up' to the boss are not in her social toolbox, and this can cause others to dislike her socially, despite her being skilled at her job.

> My tolerance for insincere people is very low as well as my ability to take everyone's case on board and fight their battles. Unfairness is probably my main hurdle. My complete honesty and bluntness don't seem to be an attribute in climbing the career ladder.

> I would really struggle with perceived pointless rules that employers had.

Gender expectations at work

There are specific situations in some workplaces where women are generally expected to take on certain roles without question. Autistic women may not naturally step into these roles or even know that it is expected of them. We are often gender-blind in this respect and expect everyone to be treated equally, not seeing invisible gender expectations of tea-making for visitors, gift-buying for colleagues' new babies and general gossip. Even if these roles are explained, it is likely that an autistic woman would question their validity or reject them in a direct manner, potentially causing herself to be seen as 'difficult'.

> Of course, being a woman, I was born knowing how to make the perfect cup of tea or coffee [...] However, what they don't bank on is my rubbish short-term memory [...] by the time I've reached the kitchen I've forgotten the ratio of coffee : tea : milk : sugar.

> Multi-tasking is a major expectation of women in workplaces. Doing all the things at once while smiling and chatting. When I tell people I can't do that, they think I am joking or making a political point. I'm really not.

> I never understood why it was rude to not let people know I was going to the shop, often putting myself under extra stress to remember to ask, 'does anyone want anything from the shop?' and then try and remember what they asked for / be able to find said item that I don't normally buy.

> Apparently, it should be expected that women make drinks / go to lunch together so they can chat, when I was looking forward to some time alone!

Disclosure and adjustments

> I have made the decision to be open about my autism in the workplace. I know that this will mean that some people make assumptions about me, but I think it's really important for there to be autistic women being visibly successful and open about who they are.

Steph Jones, autistic therapist, set up the Autism Professionals Network – which now has over 3000 followers on Instagram – to change perspectives of autistic people in their working lives. She found a surprising number of autistic women working in the caring professions, many of whom were too frightened to disclose being autistic to their employers. Steph says that this is because within mental health services, autistic people are only seen at the point of crisis as a client or patient, and the idea that the clinician may be autistic is just too great a shift for some to take.

Disclosing a disability should result in adjustments being made to accommodate that condition. Disability and equality laws differ from country to country, but this is beyond the scope of this book. Information on the rights of disabled employees should be sought from relevant sources in order to ensure that legal obligations are met by employers. Many women choose not to disclose their autism spectrum disorder (ASD) to employers for fear of discrimination, as not all employers are open to supporting staff to perform to their optimum capability.

> I have been talked to and treated in ways I don't perceive happens with other people, including being treated exploitatively. I've been neither offered accommodations or adjustments or any kind of specific support, and at times I have felt I was being punished for being autistic... I have been refused promotion, despite others who are not nearly as qualified or experienced as I am being promoted all around me.

> Diversity seems to stop at physical (dis)ability, race and gender within the workplace, and even then many fall short. Until corporate companies offer all employees, as an absolute bare minimum, the option of working in their own / a dedicated quiet room or in an open office, or working from home as a standard part of employment, regardless of any pay grade, I don't see how autism is ever really included within diversity measures.

> I've been told to let people know if I need support. In reality, trying to explain what I need or advocate for those needs feels like I'd need to put in more effort than I'd benefit in potential pay-off, so I haven't bothered.

> I have not been able to acquire the accommodations that I need in the work environment. In fact, asking for accommodations has usually angered my employers, who don't understand me, don't understand autism and actually seem to resent my asking.

> There are no adjustments available when self-employed – the market is a level playing field. I have to manage my own needs

> and turn traits into strengths and my strengths, into what I offer my clients.

> I actually don't need much support or many accommodations to thrive in the workplace or to do my job well. But I do need people to understand that when I say 'I find filling in forms really difficult, please help me' or 'I can't follow that list of instructions unless it's written down'... I really mean it. I will give it a go, but I will make mistakes and I will get highly stressed, and as a result I am likely to get ill and need time off work.

When disclosure is received positively and adjustments are made either by others or themselves – often quite small ones – autistic women can achieve success at work and maintain their well-being.

> I do receive support and adjustments – I don't have to go to conferences or do public speaking, and people weren't allowed to move my desk without a lot of warning and consultation when reorganizing the office. I am very open about having an ASC [autism spectrum condition] at work, and that takes the pressure off me as I don't have to pretend so much to be something I'm not.

> On a few occasions people in charge of me would write instructions down or try to make them easier to understand, and I appreciated this a great deal.

> I have now found a role where I've developed confidence in my abilities because I receive positive feedback. People appreciate my attention to detail, and I enjoy repetitive routine tasks that other people don't seem to like doing, e.g. filing, categorizing, routine correspondence, setting up systems, proofreading. I work hard, and I work all the hours I am paid to. I only chat to colleagues if they initiate it, and I don't go for cigarette breaks or stand around the water cooler gossiping, or whatever you're supposed to do when you work in an office!

> People have tried to push me into more growth (of my business), but since I discovered I am autistic (in 2018) I have decided that that would not be beneficial for me or my customers.

> Working from home is good for me as I can manage my energy levels and take breaks without needing to communicate or being interrupted.

> I work far fewer hours but on a month-to-month basis achieve at least as much as my peers. I have had to learn to recognize, work with and respect my individual patterns of and needs for focus, daydreaming and switching off completely. I am slow to learn new skills and slow to write, but I am thorough and systematic in the way that I work, which saves hours of wasted time.

> As much as my mask allows me to carry out the [fitness coaching] session effectively, it exhausts me, so I leave an hour between appointments when most therapists do back-to-back appointments.

Ideal job

Considering the difficulties of employment for autistic women, I was interested in knowing how these women felt they would perform best. Self-employment, part-time working, home-working and working alone featured most frequently in the responses of the women questioned. There was no mention of earning large incomes or achieving a high-status career position. It appears that spending their days doing something that does not exceed limitations is the priority for these women. Many facets of their ideal job choices mirror my own working life, which I have whittled into something that I can just about manage and have continued to whittle as my capacity decreases with age. I am self-employed, spend most of my days alone, have no ongoing daily social relationships to maintain and get to take as much time off as I wish (with the accompanying lack of income). I have no ambition beyond financial survival, maintaining interest in my work and remaining well. Other women expressed their own requirements.

> [...] Flexible part-time hours. Two reasons for this: one is because physically I get exhausted having to interact with people for long periods of time and need a quiet place and solitude to recharge my batteries. Second, I need to have time to pursue my own interests outside work because, again, this is how I re-energize myself and reduce my anxiety levels.

> I have had several ideal jobs. I loved teaching music. I loved nutrition coaching. I love my current research and delivering workshops. I thrive in roles where I can blend creative processes, efficient systems and educating other people to help make positive and beneficial change.

One woman had some much more specific job roles in mind:

> [...] Ideal job would be something involving the Discworld – either creatively or at the Discworld Emporium shop in Wincanton. Failing that, then working in or owning an independent bookshop (specializing in sci-fi/fantasy – maybe like the Forbidden Planet bookshops in London), [an] animal sanctuary (Monkey World in Dorset, or one involving donkeys, dogs, or otters or other marine life), or some sort of environmental conservation (woodlands or coastal) or a nursery (for plants, not children!).

My own autism and employment research (Hendrickx, 2009) found that autistic individuals are most successful in jobs that play to the strengths of their autism and minimize exposure to the differences, rather than trying to squeeze a square peg into a round hole. This seems to be confirmed by the women who responded to my questionnaire.

> I use my neurotype to my advantage, with attention to detail,

> innovative problem solving and hyper-focus fuelling my creations [fashion designer].

> I absolutely adore identifying imbalances and asymmetries that, I have been told, many other sports therapists have missed or not even done with my clients in the past. However, I can sometimes focus too much on the small details of someone's alignment rather than looking at the whole movement/picture of what's going on and what is most important for that session.

Chapter 12

EATING

JESS HENDRICKX

The whole system of eating seems like a needlessly complicated way to create really expensive poop.

Autistic woman

Personal experience with food

Food and eating are something that we have no choice but to engage in every day, several times a day. There are other things in our lives that we can avoid if they feel too overwhelming or pointless, but eating is not one of them – we need to eat to survive. There are multiple elements to each mealtime, such as decision-making, planning, shopping, preparing, consuming and cleaning up. For autistic people who have difficulties with any one of these things, every time they eat adds an additional load.

My professional interest in autism and eating started when I studied my postgraduate certificate (PGC) in autism in 2021. When deciding on what my theme would be, I noticed a distinct lack of information and research on the topic of how autistic adults' eating habits may differ from the neurotypical population, which, I must admit, baffled me. As an autistic woman myself, I wondered why most of the research seemed to be focused on children. This is also the case with published books. After all, being autistic is lifelong, and so is the need to eat. It is almost like researchers seem to forget that autistic people grow up just like non-autistic people do! Due to the lack of research on how autistic people interact with food, I decided to complete my PGC on autism and clinical eating disorders, specifically anorexia nervosa.

I work as a mentor with autistic adults and also as a non-clinical autism assessor. Food/eating is something that comes up quite regularly in sessions and assessments. I am not a dietician or nutritionist, but I try to help my clients to find easy solutions to their eating challenges. This normally involves coming up with quick and easy ways for them to cook and organize food, and also thinking of ways to prompt them to eat at all.

My own relationship with food did not start off particularly smoothly. As a small – unbeknown to my parents – autistic child, I was an incredibly picky eater. There were times that I lived on tinned hotdogs and spaghetti hoops and refused to eat anything else – healthy! From what I have been told, mealtimes were a constant battle. I would change my mind about liking/not liking certain vegetables on a daily basis and had a very restricted diet. That being said, when I had foods in front of me that I enjoyed I had more than a healthy appetite (I grew out of kids' size meal portions in restaurants from about the age of five). As mentioned, back then my mother did not know I was autistic, but looking back at my relationship with food and thinking about it now, it makes sense. As I got older, I became more adventurous with food, and now it is a massive part of my life. However, there are things, such as fresh tomatoes and raw onion, that ruin meals for me and can cause me to physically retch.

I still have fixed routines with foods. At the weekend I plan evening meals for the coming week, and I have set go-to meals for breakfast and lunch. If dinner plans change or my go-to foods are not available, I can struggle to know what to eat and then become overwhelmed with all of the possible options. This results in me snacking on crisps and biscuits or buying takeaways for dinner. I have a busy household of up to six mouths to feed, and I try to keep the meals as varied as possible, but we do end up eating very similar things each week. Even though I love food and cooking, I struggle to have the motivation to cook after a day at work and dealing with the kids. If I am just feeding myself, efficiency and taste are the key to my decision-making.

Like a lot of autistic women, I also have some problems with interoception (the ability to recognize those internal feelings such as hunger or thirst). If I am focused on a task, I have been known to forget to eat. It is only when I get to the point of feeling sick, shaky or dizzy that I will remember that I have not consumed anything but coffee and water all day. On the flip side, if I am eating something I love I will eat until I feel sick. I can't win!

Food to me is not just fuel. It brings me joy, governs my whole life and therefore could probably be described as an intense interest. I get very annoyed if I can't eat what I want when I want. When finding out that I was gluten intolerant a few years ago, it felt like the worse thing in the world. The thought of never again eating KFC filled me with dread. And even though gluten makes me balloon and feel awful, I do give in to urges occasionally.

When writing this chapter, my suspicions about how important the way autistic women and girls eat were confirmed. My personal opinion is that society is very quick to pathologize everything to do with autism, which leads people to feel alienated and alone. We should be embracing differences rather than scorning them, and I hope that this chapter helps people not to feel as alone in the world.

What's food got to do with autism?

Everything! From the research I have conducted and the autistic women and girls I have met throughout my life, eating differences and autism go hand in hand. And there is a very logical reason for this...

Let's first take a look at the diagnostic criteria for autism. In a nutshell, autistic women and girls have:

- a need for sameness, structure and routines
- hyper- or hyposensitive sensory differences
- social interaction and communication differences.

Although food is not explicitly mentioned, each one of the criteria can change how autistic females eat and interact with food. For example, being autistic explains: why someone might need to eat at the same time of day or use the same plate (structure/routine); their strong likes and dislikes of food based on their textures, tastes and/or smells (sensory); or how they struggle to eat in front of other people (social). These are only three potential eating needs that being autistic explains, and in this chapter I will be looking into these areas and more, and how being autistic contributes to them.

As we know, being autistic is lifelong. Our preferences with food may change over time, and also appear more or less rigid, but autism has an impact on how autistic people eat throughout their whole life. In adults, this may not be quite as obvious to other people, as when we are adults we have more control over what, when and how we eat. We can also find ways to meet our own needs rather than being reliant on someone else getting it 'right' for us. This may go some way to explaining why most research is focused on the eating differences of autistic children as generally they do not have as much say in what there is to eat.

In this chapter I will be discussing:

- sensory eating – taste, smell, textures and brands
- structures, systems and routines – how food is eaten, when food is eaten and what food is eaten with
- the impact of eating outside of the home
- clinical eating disorders – anorexia nervosa, pica and avoidant restrictive food intake disorder (ARFID).

In the years I have been a mentor, I have not met an autistic person who does not describe some sort of personal difference with regards to their relationship with food and drink. When conducting research for this chapter, I spoke to 17 autistic women and the mothers of three autistic girls about how being autistic affects how they eat and their relationship with food. The ages of these people range from 5 to 68 years of age. The majority are based in the UK with one in the US. One woman has a learning disability and one anorexia nervosa. I have tried to show as broad a selection of eating habits and preferences as possible. The majority of these women told of how they had clear preferences on the types of foods they favoured. These foods are mainly influenced by strong likes and dislikes of certain textures. They also commented on how having systems and routines for how and when they ate helped them, along with the crockery and cutlery they used. Even though everyone has their own particular likes and dislikes, which can differ from one person to another, the commonality is the existence and the strength of these women's preferences.

But it is not just about the food itself. Most of the autistic women I spoke with had varying degrees of difficulty when eating outside of the home (at school, at friends'/family's houses or in a restaurant). The most common problems were to do with environmental sensory input (mainly noise levels) and social expectations.

Autism and eating research review

There seems to be a lack of specific research on how autistic women and girls interact with food. The majority of research is focused on eating disorders, eating differences in children, those with learning disabilities or not female specific (Schröder, Danner, Spek and Elburg, 2022). In conducting my research, what stuck out to me is that most research uses language such as 'eating disturbances' and 'disordered eating' and does not focus on how the diverse ways autistic people eat may actually benefit them. Of the research that has been conducted on autism and eating (not eating disorders), the majority is not gender specific. A 2021 article by Petitpierre, Luisier and Bensafi looked into existing research on how the senses can affect the eating patterns of autistic children (not female specific). They found that neophobia (an adverse reaction to new stimuli including food) was common, as was having strict preferences for particular brands of food and a refusal of foods based on texture alone.

The first published article on autism and eating disorders was in 1983 by Christopher Gillberg. Gillberg had seen a similarity between autism and anorexia nervosa. He compared his male autistic patients to their family members who were anorexic. Since then there has been a fair amount of research into the links between autism and anorexia nervosa due to the overlaps in traits such as rigidity, social differences and sensory differences (e.g. Baron-Cohen *et al.*, 2013; Oldershaw *et al.*, 2011). Autism and eating disorders will be discussed in more depth later in this chapter. Even though there are many different clinical eating disorders, I will cover anorexia nervosa, pica and ARFID as these are the eating disorders most commonly experienced by autistic women and girls. According to research by Råstam (2008), some of the other eating disorders associated with autism are neophobia (fear of trying new foods), polydipsia (over-consumption of water to an intoxicating level), overeating and selective eating (eating ten different foods or fewer). When conducting my own research, there was once again a lack of information on the eating disorders mentioned by Råstam and how they may affect autistic people in particular. It appeared that the research conducted focused on, and included, participants from the non-autistic population.

Autistic eating

Sensory eating

As mentioned earlier on in this chapter, the sensory aspect of food appears to be the most important. Autistic women and girls have a whole range of different sensory needs in general. These can include being hypersensitive to (needing less of) or hyposensitive to (needing more of) light, touch, smells, noise and taste/textures of foods. All sensory differences are lifelong, but autistic women report that these can vary throughout their lives and can also be influenced by different situations.

The senses play a big part when it comes to eating. What food looks like, feels like in both the hand and mouth, smells like and tastes like all influence how we eat. Everyone, autistic or not, has likes and dislikes, and they all differ. However, within the autistic population these likes/dislikes appear to be much stronger. It is important to remember that it is not the preference of a particular texture/taste/smell/sight that is significant but that there is a strong preference to the point were certain food items will be avoided or sought out.

Interestingly, most women I spoke with did not report strong likes/dislikes to foods based on smells or tastes alone. One said that they do not eat olives due to the smell, and another mentioned that she hated the smell of liver, kidneys and mushy peas. One mother reported that her daughter 'hates cheese as it's a weird texture and can have a strong smell', but texture does also feature in why she does not like it.

With regards to tastes, one woman told of how she seeks out spicy foods so hot that they make her cry:

> I would eat food that is almost unbearably and dangerously spicy. There are periods of time when I enjoy crying while eating because the dish is so hot. It's rare to find a pepper that hot in the UK and all chillies taste mild to me, and I will sometimes develop a mild depression that specifically relates to chasing heat.

And another, of how she makes food taste better regardless of what others think:

> I have ketchup on everything except eggs because generally it makes it much more tasty for me. I love soggy sausage rolls done in the microwave then smoked paprika on top. It's gorgeous to me, but people say it's rank and I'm strange.

Apart from these, what was most commonly reported was how the texture of foods affected the enjoyment they got from them and how important it is that it is right. There do seem to be some textures that are more commonly desired. Crunchy foods seem to be favoured by a lot of women and girls.

> I seek out foods that are hard, dry, crispy and easy to eat. Examples of this are crisps, cheese and snack-based food that I can pick up with fingers.

> I very actively seek out dry, crunchy food. I had to abandon a low-carb diet because very few low-carb foods are crunchy (anybody who tells me nuts and carrots are crunchy can bugger off).

However, it is not always crunchy food that people veer towards; others reported seeking out softer or mushy textures of food.

> [I] seek out soft, mushy, wet, mashed [food], covered in gravy. Mashed potato, porridge, custard, milk puddings, tinned macaroni cheese, Greek yogurt, cream, Angel Delight, squirty cream, Weetabix with enough milk to break down the texture to a mush, shepherd's pie, fish pie.

The texture of foods that are sought may also depend on mood. Someone I met once said that she seeks out soft foods when she is tired as they take less effort to eat. It is clear to see the variety of textures that autistic women and girls enjoy, but what textures do they avoid? The most mentioned was slimy, stodgy and lumpy foods, especially mashed potatoes.

> I avoid foods that are slimy or lumpy. I hate lumpy mashed potato. I use a ricer to make it smooth.

> I can struggle with lumpy food that isn't supposed to be lumpy, e.g. mashed potatoes; I cannot eat slimy foods as I gag.

> [My daughter] avoids lumpy foods and stodgy foods such as mashed potatoes, rice and pasta, which can be too wet and soft. (Parent)

The texture of dry, over-cooked meat was remarked on by two women who both had difficulties in swallowing them.

> [...] Avoid dry meat like roast beef. As a child I couldn't swallow chunks of chewed meat, couldn't eat liver – too dry.

> I hate things that are overdone. I have to have things underdone like bacon or chicken, etc. If anything comes to me that is hard like bacon, especially if it's crispy, I send it back as it makes it hard for me to swallow it to the point that it makes me feel sick [...] I could go on but you would need a new book to put it in.

It appears that the texture of foods can override the taste. If the texture is wrong, a food item may not be consumed, regardless of whether or not someone likes the taste of it.

> Texture is enormously important to me. I cannot cope with the rubbery texture of mushrooms, they make me physically start retching; but if I purée mushrooms then they're fine – which tells me it's not about the flavour at all.

> The texture is more important than taste. If I don't like the texture it completely changes how it tastes.

Autistic women and girls obviously have preferences when it comes to texture and taste, but that does not wholly explain why some may have limited diets. Choosing foods due to the predictability of them is another reason for this. Let's think about apples and how unpredictable they can be. It does not matter what colour, shape or size; no one apple ever tastes the same. There are so many variants, but you cannot tell just by looking at it. The texture could be all wrong: it might be too juicy, too sour or too sweet – and the only way to tell is by biting into it. And this is the case with so many other foods, especially most fruit and some vegetables.

> [My daughter] seeks out easy foods [such as] crackers, bread sticks, chips; she keeps to things that she knows won't change so no surprises, e.g. fruit changes colour and texture. (Parent)

> I am generally okay with most types of food textures, as long as that is how the food is supposed to taste/feel like. For example, I like the mushy texture of soup, but mashed banana makes me gag. I like crunching on raw vegetables, but if a piece of fruit is crunchy because it's unripe then I won't eat it.

> The foods that I like are my comfort zone. I feel very safe when eating them, especially chocolate.

> I find I seek out foods that are dry, either hard or soft, but not both at the same time as the texture has to be consistent. This is both how it feels in my mouth and dealing with having to hold it.

The shock of finding something that was not expected can ruin the whole thing. This aversion to unpredictability in foods and things not being right can cause autistic women to leave whole meals.

> I like meat and fish, but if I find any gristle or bones when I'm eating it then I don't enjoy the rest of the meal as I am focusing too much on each mouthful in case of other bits that shouldn't be there. Sometimes I'll leave the whole meal if it's particularly bad.

Favouring specific brands for certain foods also alleviates some of the uncertainty. There may be small variations in taste, size and texture from one brand to another, and these are very noticeable to some. Interestingly, brand preference appears to be more important in childhood than adulthood. The brand name is not the important aspect; it is solely based on the taste and texture compared to other brands.

> [My daughter] can tell the difference between brands, e.g. will eat breaded chicken fingers by McCain but not battered chicken as the texture is wrong. (Parent)

> As a child I was instantly able to tell the difference between a

> variety of tinned foods, such as baked beans or spaghetti. The subtle difference made it impossible to eat the food, I think, because I was not expecting it and it became a forced transition – with time I may have been able to but not otherwise.

> I've always been very aware of different brands and can tell between own brands of foods and official brands. These would include most cereals, most noticeably in Shreddies and Coco Pops. Different types of sauces are clear for me from the different taste of condiments like mayonnaise and ketchup to the sauce in baked beans. [...] I grew up having own-brand versions of food so having official brands tastes like a different food sometimes completely. There have been times when I've thought the food was off because the different taste has been so different, especially if I wasn't expecting it.

> It was particularly important as a child; every brand had to be the right one.

If you are the parent of an autistic girl, I would recommend not trying to trick her into eating an alternative, as apparently it does not work!

> Other brands tasted wrong, stale, incorrect, uncomfortable; it felt like I was eating a totally different food – and that would probably have been okay if I hadn't been expecting it to be the thing I was familiar with. My parents even tried switching out boxes of cereal because they thought I wouldn't notice if it was in the right box, but I always did.

This shows very clearly that it has nothing to do with the packaging and everything to do with the product itself. What is interesting about this woman's experience is that it is the surprise that appears to be the issue, and if given prior warning, then it may not have posed as much of a problem for her. However, this is not the case for everyone. At times, brands discontinue items or shops run out.

For some this can cause a lot of anxiety, an inability to make decisions or a refusal to eat an alternative.

> I get very cross and very upset and frustrated if I can't find the food that I like to eat. It's really hard when it's not in stock especially; it makes shopping harder for me too.

> She would choose not to eat at all if an alternative acceptable food was not available. She benefits from the consistency of the same brands. (Parent)

> This has been a problem on occasions when foods have been discontinued. If I have warning of the discontinuation, I will buy as many as I can to give me time to find something else. This has been very difficult if I have no warning and I am then left stuck in the supermarket for hours trying to find something that feels acceptable, but it's very hard to let go of the food I feel safe with. Every time the result in finding an alternative has meant I've replaced the food with a much lower [calorie] option as restriction makes me feel like I'm back in control.

> If the brand is not available, she would leave the food given and not even try and eat it as she will say it looks and smells funny. (Parent)

Structure, systems and routines

Now that we have a bit more of an understanding of and insight into how important the sensory aspects of food are to autistic women and girls, I will outline what part structures, systems and routines play. As we know, following strict routines and having systems in all areas of one's life are common for autistic women and girls. These routines provide a sense of security and calm in a mostly chaotic world. I know many autistic women who meticulously plan out every aspect of their days, weeks, months and years, and what and when they eat can be part of that. It makes sense that food would be part of this planning as it is something that we need to engage in multiple times each day. Preparation can alleviate the anxiety brought on from not knowing what is going to happen. Not every eventuality can be planned for, but having a safety net of predictability to fall back on can help when things suddenly become out of one's control.

When to eat is the most logical place to start. Keeping to those routines provides consistency and can help to shape the rest of one's day.

> [My daughter] sticks to a routine and will have breakfast at the same time each day; when she's not at school she will have lunch the same time and dinner is the same unless we are out, but she will still say she's hungry at the time we normally eat. (Parent)

It is clear that for this child change poses a problem and causes her to become distressed. Her mother keeping the routine the same every day helps her daughter, and in turn herself.

> We stick to these routines as change for [my daughter] can cause meltdowns. So to keep things calm we follow the same pattern. (Parent)

For some, the need for routine is more to do with the physical effect that eating at the wrong time can have. What is particularly interesting about this next quote is why having fixed routines benefits her and what happens if she cannot stick to them:

> I have to eat at 11 a.m. and eat at 5 p.m. (no later), as if I do, it gives me terrible sleep and indigestion and it makes me feel sick and anxious [...] sticking to my routine makes me feel better and happier about myself. If that routine is changed in any way, boy oh boy, watch out.

Another aspect of eating structures is not just when you eat but how. This can include factors such as how food is arranged on the plate, the order in which it is consumed, and what crockery, cup and cutlery are used. Just like in Michelin-starred restaurants, how food is presented matters a lot. Cross-contamination for some autistic women and girls is a no-go. Having food separate on the plate is important.

> [My daughter] uses a divided plate so that no food touches another and has more picky foods, as she can struggle with cutlery as she finds it hard to hold and use. If unavailable she has food on a plate separately (still not touching) or we do a picnic with her lunchbox as this is less pressure on her. (Parent)

> [...] Food item must not be touching, most easily achieved by separate bowls. As [my daughter's] anxiety is decreasing after withdrawing from school she can tolerate infringements into this method of eating. (Parent)

> I can eat most things, but if something that was meant to be dry and crunchy touched another food that made it wet and soggy, I would be disproportionately upset even now at 43.

Interestingly, this need was also mentioned by two adult autistic women about two specific food items – eggs and baked beans.

> Some things make me feel queasy, e.g. egg touching bean.

> I hate baked beans on or near my eggs, it makes me very cross.

This is something that I wholeheartedly agree with. I must admit, I hadn't realized this was a thing until I read these responses and had always believed it was one of those 'I thought it was just me' things!

Even though no one that contributed to this chapter mentioned it, I do know of autistic women who like to have certain meals completely mixed up together. These meals tend to just have two elements to them, one of them being wet, the other dry (e.g. rice and curry, or pasta and sauce), and not something like a roast dinner. Their reason for mixing them together is so that each spoonful is as consistent as possible which therefore limits surprises.

When I asked autistic women about the order that they eat their food it became clear that having a system for this is also essential and added to their enjoyment of their meal or lessened the stress at mealtimes. Saving the best bit to last seemed to be quite a common. This makes sense to me, as the last taste is then the best bit! Just as with textures and tastes, the important thing is not the system itself but the fact that there is a system at all. These autistic women and girls are clearly making a very conscious effort to eat in a very particular way.

> I'll eat everything I don't like first; I'll eat one thing at a time (e.g. not meat, veg and potatoes in the same mouthful); I'll very deliberately save a particular piece of whatever I'm eating to eat last, the best piece.

> From when I was very young, I've always had a system that I still use today. I eat the thing I enjoy the least, and then move towards the thing that I enjoy the most. I used to be stricter with this when I was a child, eating all my peas first, followed by my potato, then finishing with the meat.

> I manage the amount of each item on my plate/bowl to ensure that none run out before any of the others. I do not like single flavours and textures of foods and like to create planned fork/spoonfuls which have a mix of a number of different foods.

> If I'm eating a hot dinner, I usually have a little bit of everything in each mouthful.

If these systems are interrupted the reaction can be strong to say the least!

> Nothing makes me angrier than somebody coming along and taking a sweet from me whilst I'm in the middle of eating them, especially if it's one that I've been saving for the grand finale! It makes me very angry if someone takes something from me

> without asking first. If they ask, I give them the one that is the least desirable.

> If for example my partner were to 'steal' the piece of potato I'd been saving for last I'd be very upset, possibly tearful.

Making sure that mealtimes are as stress free as possible is incredibly important and these systems can aid in this.

> It doesn't really [benefit me] other than creating a sense of calm and order and control. Meals can be a break from the stress of a day, or they can add to it.

Not having to make conscious decisions about how they eat helps autistic women and girls to focus solely on the food and their enjoyment of it. This also highlights how important routines are in all aspects of autistic females lives. One woman talked of, 'my love of routine I suppose. Also, you don't have to make choices'.

Consistency is not just reflected in when and how autistic women and girls eat but also with what crockery and cutlery. Personally, I prefer particular mugs, at different times of the day and depending on what hot drink I am having. My partner will ask me which one I want if he makes me a drink as he understands the importance of this for me. If it is not served in the correct one, this takes away from some of the enjoyment due to it not being right, and I am not alone in this thought process.

> Mugs – I have to have big mugs, I can't cope with small mugs; they don't give you enough to drink, whereas with big mugs you get lots more in it. Also I like eating with a dessert spoon and fork – weird I know but that's what I do. Yes, I see people stare at me in restaurants like I'm strange, but oh well.

It does not stop at mugs and drinks. Having the correct cutlery and crockery also has an impact on one's enjoyment of food. I recently bought new plates and I have discovered that food looks and tastes better when I use the light purple or blue ones, and I refuse to use the peach-coloured ones. I am putting this down to the preference of colour alone. Why would I eat off something that I do not like the colour of? I would be preoccupied by the fact that I do not like the colour, and that would take away from the joy of what I am eating. Other autistic women have similar needs.

> [...] Same spoon, fork, plate, bowl (well three bowls: one for cereal/stew, one for lunch noodles and a huge one for big portions of soup). They're just 'right': there's something comforting and reassuring from a sensory point of view, I know what they look and feel like [...] I've had the same plate for 26 years. I'm not overly anxious about dropping it (although I make great efforts not to) as I will be able to find another 'right' plate; it's more about predictability and a sense of ease when I can use the same crockery/cutlery – it's one less thing in my day that takes extra energy.

> I always eat my food in a bowl and with a spoon. I have preferences for certain spoons and other cutlery and will deliberately avoid others. I use different bowls and plates for different meals and types of foods, but this is according to a fixed set of rules. I cut my food into small enough pieces to be eaten with a spoon only.

If a preferred item of crockery or cutlery is not available, then this can have quite a substantial impact on mealtimes.

> It makes me feel very uncomfortable and sad, but I eventually get over it after three hours.

> I would not enjoy my food and would be distracted by thinking about how wrong it is.

Eating in an unconventional way

Culturally, we eat certain things at certain times of the day. This can vary from country to country, but any deviations from the norms would likely be frowned upon, wherever you are in the world. In the UK, it is common to have cereal, toast or a fry-up for breakfast, sandwiches or soup for lunch, and some mix of protein, carbs and veg for dinner. In my opinion these are just silly, arbitrary rules. Why can't we eat whatever we want, at whatever time of day we want it? We can, and we should, regardless of other people's judgement!

> I have a ham sandwich every day for breakfast, don't really do lunch – never see the point. Dinner I have at 5 p.m.; that's normally chicken stew, etc.

> I have been known to order chips as a dessert because I don't like/want the traditional sweet options. I was laughed at for this, but I did enjoy them!

> I do love breakfast for dinner. I thought everyone likes that. I like coffee at night. Everyone does, right?

Just like when we eat certain foods, non-traditional flavour combinations are also frowned upon.

> Porridge with black treacle, banana and Greek yogurt raised a few eyebrows from my family. Peanut butter and jam, jam and cheese: I like the combination of sweet and savoury. So pancakes with bacon and maple syrup is yummy!

> I put sauces on things that some people find weird [...] I dip fries in ice-cream. I put orange juice on toast. Things like that. Sugar in sour cream.

We may not agree with what or how someone is eating, but if it is not harming them, let's just leave them be to have fun with food and eat in their own unique way. Obviously, as varied a diet as possible is the healthiest option, but if this can be achieved by using the same crockery and cutlery every mealtime and eating curry for breakfast, I would throw caution to the wind and embrace it.

Preparing/planning foods

The sensory aspects of food, and how routines, structures and systems can impact the way autistic women and girls eat and interact with food, are incredibly important but what influence does the autistic brain have on planning what to eat and then preparing the food? Apparently, quite a lot!

> It varies depending on how exhausted I am and how important it is that I do it. So I can cook a three-course Christmas dinner if I need to, but sometimes can eat cereal for two days in a row as I can't decide what to cook, or all the steps needed to make a meal are too much. Some days even getting the right vegetable out of the fridge seems too hard.

What's important to note is that what has happened throughout the day influences how able an autistic woman is to prep and cook food. Dr Luke Beardon illustrates how the environment can have both a positive and negative impact on autistic people with his equation: Autism + Environment = Outcome (Beardon, 2017). The environment is not limited to someone's physical surroundings but also how they feel internally (e.g. how tired or hungry they are). Taking external and internal factors into account when planning and preparing food can aid in the ease of carrying out such tasks. For example, if a day is looking particularly busy, plan to have either something easy that requires no thought or a takeaway. Try to make life as hassle free as possible. Another way to do this is to stick to similar meals each week that use up a smaller amount of energy.

> We have a lot of the same meals each week because I find meal planning quite difficult, so I buy the same shopping and cook roughly the same food, maybe doing something different on a Saturday when I have more head space.

Multiple input can cause the autistic brain to become overwhelmed very quickly. Factoring this in when cooking is important. Linking back to Dr Luke Beardon's equation, if the environment is right, the outcome is likely to be better.

> I take a very long time to cook, so usually double the time it says on the recipe. I can't do things concurrently, so I have to prepare all the ingredients before I start cooking; I couldn't be chopping veg whilst the meat is frying as I can't concentrate on two things. I need everyone else to stay out of the kitchen whilst I'm cooking and not talk to me, particularly when I'm dealing with hot things as I'm liable to burn myself.

Eating out of the home

From memory, most school dinners were not the most pleasant of experiences! I am sure that we all remember the joys of blanc-mange, over-boiled frozen mixed veg, grey bits of meat, instant mashed potato and milk that tasted sour. The difficulties autistic girls may face when having lunches in the school canteen are not only due the food itself. Canteens are loud, echoey, over-lit spaces – a sensory nightmare. There is the social element to contend with as well.

> I used to have great difficulty with school dinners as a young child, so much so that I always went home for lunch until secondary school. Then I usually took the same packed lunch every day for seven years, with occasional school dinners.

> [My daughter] struggled to eat at school due to noise in the lunch hall; she now wears ear defenders and sits away from school dinners, which has helped. (Parent)

As we grow up and move away from school life and enter adulthood, there are more pressures to eat away from the house. The sensory element of eating in a restaurant is a very real problem, especially when somewhere is very busy. For the women who contributed to this book, noise seemed to be the biggest sensory issue. From conducting non-clinical assessments, I have noticed that having multiple inputs of noise is something a lot of autistic women and girls can struggle with (background music, chatter of other people, children, chairs scraping, etc.).

> It's very hard as I'm extremely sensitive to noise [...] I don't like eating out if I can help it; drink wise I'm good but not eating as I feel like everyone is staring at me and talking about me. I get very uncomfortable and uneasy.

> I enjoy eating out, I like food and I like not having to cook but find noise/lighting/people sitting too close or walking too close to the back of my chair hard. I tend to avoid eating out in a group as several conversations happening at once is too much; eating out with one other person and either early when it's quiet or on a weeknight can be enjoyable, although I usually get anxious beforehand about getting there on time. Also, I always try and let the other person walk into the restaurant first so I don't have to cope with the overload of lights/noise/people at the same time as navigating to a table without banging into things and the horror of the waiter asking me a question.

Whether in restaurants or at other people's houses, eating out is meant to be an enjoyable, social event, but unfortunately this is not the case for some autistic women. The communication aspect combined with sensory differences can make eating in a restaurant a difficult experience for autistic women and girls.

> I don't like having to talk and eat at the same time. It makes conversation so difficult. Also because of the noise and other people who I don't know, it can make me feel anxious, which suppresses my appetite. I can rarely finish a starter and main course. By the time the main course arrives, my appetite has all but disappeared. Also, noise makes it hard to listen to what the person I am with is saying. So negotiating conversation whilst eating and struggling to hear is really hard! I cope with this by preferring quieter venues. If there is a group of people, I may go

> quiet whilst I am eating, joining in with the conversation when I have finished and the pressure has eased.

One of the most common first-date scenarios is a meal out. There is an awful lot to contend with in this situation – the social element, along with making sure you make a good first impression and having to multi-task in a busy environment.

> Having a first date with someone and going for a meal is terrifying! All of those things to negotiate, whilst getting to know someone, watching my own behaviours, trying to eat whilst struggling to finish my food, look friendly and hear what they're saying. I feel my heart rate rising just thinking about it!

Having to navigate all the aspects of eating outside of the home can be incredibly exhausting. Having coping mechanisms in place can help regardless of age or a situation that is overwhelming. This can range from choosing what to eat to limiting the impact of the sensory environment, to making sure you have time before and after to prep/recover.

> I cancel any other usual plans I have so that eating out is the *only* thing I do that day. I used to have to cancel plans the day(s) before and after too, but as it's now rare that I am forced out of my safe environments, my ability to cope and recover is better.

> When we go out, we go to the same places [my daughter] knows and have fidget toys and the iPad available to help calm her as well as ordering her favourite food to keep her happy. (Parent)

When eating away from the home, foods that are normally deemed 'safe' all of a sudden can become problematic.

> I have found many coping mechanisms to manage my eating – I will rarely let anyone cook for me because I like things cooked a certain way. I have learned that people are very sensitive if you

> refuse to eat what they have cooked, even if I have given them info on how I would like it prepared, no matter how politely I try to tell them.

I have met a lot of autistic women who look at the menu in advance (which is something I also do myself) or stick to their safe foods. Doing either of these things takes away some of the stress of having to decide in an unfamiliar environment and also the unknowns of what will be available to eat, both of which strategies can make the experience of eating out a much more pleasant one.

> I get completely overwhelmed by choosing food on a menu. I will often try and do this online before I leave home. I try to consider every possible variable that I might have – can I cook it myself? does it have carbs? am I trying to lose weight? will it make me sleepy? what else have I eaten today? will it be homemade? etc. I get so overwhelmed trying to choose the exact right thing, that I end up choosing the same thing as I have every time if it is available – Caesar salad and chips!

> I now find restaurants not very enticing, a combination of too busy and noisy, and I like to stick to my preferred foods so a big menu is off-putting, and I will often go for something very familiar such as fish and chips. Too much choice in any situation can throw me.

> [My daughter's] difficulties in decision-making affect her enjoyment of food and eating socially with friends. When eating out she does not eat what arrives despite choosing it, because it is not how she expected. (Parent)

As has been previously discussed, autistic women and girls tend to have quite fixed routines and systems in terms of how they eat and what they eat with. When in a restaurant or café, you do not have access to your own crockery and cutlery, and this can also take away some of the enjoyment of eating out.

> So, I can eat out of the house and use different cutlery/crockery, but it does add to the amount of energy I use up, albeit in a very tiny way. If a café had exactly the same style of crockery, it still wouldn't be quite the same, as their plate wouldn't have the same subtle scratches, etc., so it would still be different.

Over the last few years, being served food in weird ways has become a lot more popular. And I have no idea why!

> I hate restaurants that do not serve food in a standard plate or bowl. Having chips served in a basket, skewers hanging from a hook in front of my face or different items in separate containers are of no use to me as I need to eat my meal by combining the items. I can't cope with seeing my food in this weird, three-dimensional way. I will tip all of the items out of their vessels on to a plate. It makes me very irritated and totally unable to eat the meal until it is organized properly.

I personally have an absolute hatred of slate plates – the sound cutlery makes on them sets my teeth on edge and shivers down my spine. Restaurateurs need to stop with the silliness and just serve things in a practical way that makes them easier to eat.

Autism and eating disorders

There has been increased interest in recent years on the link between autism and eating disorders, especially within the female population and those specifically with anorexia nervosa. In this section I outline three different types of eating disorders that have been linked with autism: anorexia nervosa, avoidant restrictive food intake disorder (ARFID) and pica.

Anorexia nervosa

Anorexia nervosa is an eating disorder characterized by restricting food intake with the goal of losing weight or changing one's body shape, due to a fear of being or becoming overweight. Women with anorexia may also be suffering from body dysmorphia: seeing themselves as overweight when in fact they are underweight. There has been the suggestion too that anorexia nervosa is a form of female autism due the similarities of both conditions, which include social differences, sensory differences and a need for structure and routines (Oldershaw *et al.*, 2011; Tchanturia *et al.*, 2013).

In the UK research suggests that 20 to 30 per cent of anorexia patients are also autistic (Babb *et al.*, 2021). However, at the time of writing, there are no set guidelines on how to treat autistic women with anorexia on the NHS, meaning that a larger number of women are being treated in a way that does not work for them.

Dr Kate Tchanturia, lead clinical psychologist at the Maudsley Hospital in London, has developed the *P*athway for *E*ating *D*isorders and *A*utism Developed from *C*linical *E*xperience (PEACE), a guide for professionals on how to best support autistic people with eating disorders. There are also online resources for autistic women and their families.[1] Most research suggests that for autistic women with an eating disorder to get the best out of treatment, their support must be adapted to fit their needs (Babb *et al.*, 2021). This includes highlighting the importance of autism assessment, adapting therapies and considering the sensory differences autistic women may have both in terms of their environment and also when it comes to food textures, tastes and smells (Tchanturia, 2021)

I spoke with one woman (who I will refer to as Emma), who at the time of writing is on her fifth admission to an inpatient eating disorder unit. Emma was diagnosed with anorexia nervosa, restrictive type, at age 23 (she is now 30) and also has a previous diagnosis of obsessive-compulsive disorder (OCD) but did not feel that this quite fitted her completely.

> Looking back at my diagnosis, the psychiatrist also diagnosed me as having anankastic personality disorder or obsessive-compulsive personality disorder; it seems very interesting to me that

1 www.peacepathway.org

> she picked up what were a lot autistic traits but gave me that diagnosis instead of questioning autism itself. This was in 2015.
>
> It was picked up on my fourth admission [that] I might be autistic, and the first part of the test revealed this was the case. When needing a fifth admission, the fact I didn't have the second part of the ADOS-2 test [autism diagnostic test] and therefore in their eyes a complete diagnosis, I was forced into a lot of positions around eating that would put me in more distress.

Emma was given a full diagnosis of autism as part of her current admission. She had previously undergone the first part of the ADOS-2 (Autism Diagnostic Observation Schedule version 2) assessment, but as this had not been completed fully, Emma has struggled to access the support she needs. Only once the second part of the assessment was carried out and signed off were the team more accepting that she is autistic and may need adjustments made to her care. Due to a lack of knowledge, the specialist support Emma needs has still not been easy to get:

> Since receiving a full diagnosis, the team have struggled to understand and know the difference between my eating disorder and autism, which has in itself created a lot of issues. Changes to my treatment plan have happened but this has been a very slow process, and change only seems to happen when I've been in a prolonged state of distress, rather than my case being reviewed regularly or really looking into what adjustments can be made in order to put [in place] a plan that would suit me before I'm placed in deep distress.

Unfortunately, due to the lack of understanding and knowledge of how being autistic can have an impact on anorexia and the support that is needed when being released from inpatient care, Emma is still not able to receive the support she so desperately needs:

> In terms of [being an] outpatient, my experience has been very poor with my team stating that autism isn't their area and so

> won't be addressed in this department. It is hard to know where and who can actually support me once I become [an] outpatient but there are services that are looking into this, which is different to any of my other admissions prior to my autism diagnosis.

Emma's situation is also echoed in the Babb *et al.* (2021) study on how autistic women may find accessing the support more difficult due to being autistic. One participant in the study said, 'I think the co-existence of [autism] as well as the eating disorder is something that just makes some adults teams feel, "It's just too complicated, we just don't really want to know"' (Babb *et al.*, 2021). The go-to therapy is cognitive behavioural therapy (CBT) and group work – both of which can cause problems for autistic women.

> With the CBT, maybe the problem is that they assume you have lots of these skills already... Therefore, I couldn't even begin to make changes, because I don't have any of those foundational skills. (Autistic female participant of Babb *et al.*, 2021)

> I'm largely silent in any sort of group situation because I don't know what's expected of me. I'm worried of saying the wrong thing or I worry about misinterpreting people. (Autistic female participant of Babb *et al.*, 2021)

Why do autistic teenage girls stop eating?

The teen years are an incredibly difficult period of life for autistic females, regardless of whether they know their diagnosis or not. I remember first hand only too well how hard it was to navigate the social minefield of secondary-school life and having that overwhelming need to fit in. I was fortunate that I did not develop an eating disorder, but there are many autistic girls out there who do, and some do not get the help they need.

> I was never diagnosed with an eating disorder, but at the age of 14 I developed severely restricted eating patterns. I never received any treatment. I was feeling very out of control in my

> life, and I was very aware that being thin was perceived as being good and doing well. I was already slim, weighed about eight-and-a-half stone and was five feet eight inches, but decided that I needed to be thinner, and it would make me feel better.

For some, the goal of losing weight is not a conscious one but the result of not feeling like they were the same as their peers.

> I would have preferred to have been invisible during my teens and early twenties and made an unconscious attempt to do this when I lost an incredible amount of weight and became very underweight for a time.

Anecdotally, some autistic women report that it is during their teen years they start to really notice the differences between themselves and their peers. Their neurotypical peers start to rapidly move away from what are deemed to be more child-like interests and grow more interested in romantic relationships and gender-specific interests. The teen years are also when social relationships become more complex, and girls become much more focused on what other people think of them. During this time, it makes sense to me that autistic girls may want to control and limit their food intake, not just to lose weight and fit in, but also to feel like they have some level of control over their lives. If you assign rules to how many calories you can consume and when you can eat, this will go some way to providing a daily relief from the uncertainty in the world. However, for some girls this becomes a problem when they start to be dangerously underweight, and medical intervention is needed.

Autistic women's motivations to restrict food may differ from those of the non-autistic population. Body changes during puberty, such as menstruation and the development of breasts or a more womanly figure, may also be the catalyst for restricting their food intake. These changes in the body can cause anxiety. Malnutrition can cause menstruation to stop and the body shape to stay child-like. There is also a huge amount of pressure on women and girls to look a certain way. The media always has something to say about the 'perfect' body shape, and this may also cause autistic girls to stop eating with the hope that if they achieve these unrealistic and harmful goals they will finally be accepted.

Avoidant restrictive food intake disorder (ARFID)

ARFID is perceived as picky eating to an extreme level. There is no motivation to lose weight and it is most commonly due to sensory differences, interoception or a distinct lack of interest in eating (this can be because eating gets in the way of other tasks or activities). People with ARFID have a very limited diet in both the number of different items that they eat and the amount of food that is consumed. Even though weight loss is not a motivation, it can be very much a symptom of having such a restricted diet.

From the DSM-IV to DSM-5, ARFID has been recategorized. It was previously referred to as 'Feeding and Eating Disorders of Infancy or Early Childhood', and to be diagnosed it must have been present before six years of age. Since the revision in 2013, ARFID is no longer linked solely to children and can be onset at any age.

Pica

Pica is a compulsion to eat non-food or non-nutritive items for a period of at least one month (Schnitzler, 2022). These items may include paper, foam, coal, plastic, glass, ice and metal. At the time of writing, there has been very little research on pica and autism, especially when it comes to providing support for those with this eating disorder (Shea, Frankish and Frankish, 2019). It is thought that pica may be linked with sensory-seeking habits or potentially the body lacking certain nutrients, but with limited research it is hard to say. It does, however, make sense that engaging in pica would be to sate a sensory need. Eating non-food items in times of stress and overwhelm could potentially offer a form of comfort (Shea, Frankish and Frankish, 2019).

> I was three when the pica first started. I would eat foam from cushion and chair stuffing, and later I would eat hard plastic like that used in plastic rulers, pens, Lego and toys. I realized that

> when I chewed on and swallowed this kind of material, I felt calm and relaxed. Looking back, I can see that in school and home situations I could concentrate better and felt regulated when chewing. I liked the feeling of the materials in my mouth, and I understand now that this was an enjoyable sensory experience for me.

> I have gone through different phases of what I eat/crave, but it's usually ice/snow or oils/butter, even ones that shouldn't technically be consumed and aren't food. I actually crave it despite not being hungry. I tried to address possible causes like vitamin deficiencies, and even when supplementing for anaemia, I still have to avoid having the things I crave [around] me.

Due to the lack of information on pica and how to offer support to both parents and those with pica, punishments or deterrents were often used. However, these seldom work as the overriding need to engage in this behaviour takes over.

> My parents were terrified of the impact this behaviour would have on me. When they caught me picking and chewing, they would put sanctions in place as a punishment. Once they went to the doctor themselves but did not take me. They were given cod liver oil or castor oil to use as a deterrent or punishment. Ultimately this didn't work. When I was older, I realized the dangers associated with this behaviour and stopped. As an adult, I researched into sensory stimulation and started using sensory chews and chewlery. This gives me the same sensory feedback as pica and is safe.

A lot of the items that people seek when they have pica are not easily replicated by food items. There is nothing edible, that I can think of, that has the same texture as a plastic brick or coal. This means that trying to swap out the non-food item for something safe proves very difficult. Whether pica stems from a sensory need or lack of nutrients, the first step is to figure out why this is happening before any support can be offered.

Final thoughts

It is important to remember that every autistic person is an individual and that this chapter is just an overview. There are no wrongs or rights, and we all have our own quirks when it comes to food. If the way you eat is not harming you or others around you, I implore you to keep on doing what you're doing. Drink your coffee out of the same mug every day, but it might be a good idea to get spares if you fear what will happen if it breaks. Only eat one brand of cereal and baked beans. Put a pea on each prong of the fork if it brings you joy and makes them taste even more delicious. Refuse to eat lumpy mashed potato because it feels weird and horrible in your mouth. Only eat cheese and tomato sandwiches if it takes away any undue need to think about what to eat.

Just keep being you and remember, as one woman put it:

> I eat this way coz I'm different and unique.

Chapter 13

HEALTH AND WELL-BEING

> *I feel unwell most of the time: either a headache, stomach-ache, feelings of anxiety or general fatigue. They're nothing serious, but there's always something that means I feel less than 100 per cent. Simply existing just seems to be hard work.*
>
> Autistic woman

In this chapter, I present a sample of physical and mental health conditions and experiences most typically reported by autistic women or considered to have a connection to autism, ranging from periods to drug use and anything else in between. This is just a brief overview of some of these to share the possibility that one thing may be linked to another currently unknown thing, for which treatment or support may be available. If anything resonates, please look into research carried out by people with far greater knowledge in this area than I have. Perhaps there will be a lightbulb moment of 'Aha! That's why I have a beard / can turn my head 180 degrees / have absolutely no idea if I am sad'. Read on...

Due to the almost complete lack of research to date focusing on autistic women, the nature of any associated physical or mental health issues specific to this group is largely unknown. In my experience, and from the responses provided, it would appear that autistic women experience many different health difficulties that on the surface may appear entirely unrelated to autism, but in reality are entirely connected. Neville (2019) found that all of her participants reported physical health challenges such as digestive disorders, pain, hypermobility, migraines and autoimmunity. I have been called a hypochondriac due to my never-ending list of 'niggles', as I call them: aches, pains, intolerances and sensitivities that affect my everyday life – migraines, tinnitus, polycystic ovary syndrome (PCOS), anxiety, panic attacks, aches, insulin resistance, food intolerances, insomnia, trichotillomania, photophobia, Meares-Irlen syndrome, tics, blepharospasm... I'll stop now as it looks like I'm showing off), and I can see that the same could be said, incorrectly, of other autistic women. Some of these diagnoses preceded the diagnosis of autism and may now be understood as facets of the autism profile, rather than distinct conditions. Some are self-diagnosed, and others may be incorrect diagnoses; for example, obsessive-compulsive disorder (OCD) is sometimes wrongly diagnosed in an autistic individual when the observed behaviour is simply a need for structure and routine, rather than an irrational or compulsive thought. Obviously, how each person experiences and perceives the symptoms of these conditions varies between individuals.

> Dyslexia, dyspraxia, Meares–Irlen syndrome, generalized anxiety disorder, clinical depression, obsessive-compulsive disorder, endometriosis (severe), asthma, partially sighted, irritable bowel syndrome, Raynaud's syndrome, allergies. I think that's everything!

> Learning disabilities, dyslexia, ADD [attention deficit disorder], scotopic sensitivity syndrome (visual perceptual problems), asthma, irritable bowel syndrome (gastrointestinal issues), hypothyroidism, neuropathy, migraine disorder, depression, and anxiety disorder.

> Asthma, chronic non-allergic rhinitis, IBS [irritable bowel syndrome], ME [myalgic encephalomyelitis], migraine, synaesthesia, RSI [repetitive strain injury], chronic daytime sleepiness,

> depression (recurrent depressive disorder, I think), anxiety, PMS [premenstrual syndrome], hypoglycaemia.

> Hypermobility issues in back and neck (confirmed by chiropractic practitioner), dyscalculia (undiagnosed), depression, trichotillomania (very mild now but quite pronounced in teens, flares up with stress), generalized anxiety and eating disorder issues (under-eating and over-exercising, but not anorexia).

The impact of these conditions is undoubtedly real, and I have never yet met an autistic woman whom I believe to be fabricating their health concerns or making an unnecessary fuss. If anything, the opposite is true: these women are often just getting on with life in considerable discomfort and pain, without seeking medical help, sometimes feeling that it is 'normal' to hurt so much all of the time due to no evidence to the contrary and no peer group to ask. The hyper-awareness and detail-focused nature of an autistic person perhaps means that these women may notice more acutely when something doesn't feel right. Autistic women can turn themselves into the focus of an intense interest and become their own project. They are often experts in their own conditions and should be involved in decisions relating to any treatment process. If they do seek medical advice, it is likely that they will have researched all possible options and may even know more than the practitioner about specific conditions. Rather than become defensive about this amateur clinician, healthcare professionals would be wise to listen and take note; the woman may well be right and save the practitioner a lot of time.

> It should be [doctors'] first clue when we show up with a binder! 'What about this study? And there's this, and this?' (Neville, 2019, p.28)

> I dive in and sort of absorb all the details there are to know about a subject... There's this sort of sea of details and, out of the details, things start to come up and then they start to connect.

> You start to see the lines between the connections and then, all of a sudden, it builds up. (Neville, 2019, p.29)

It is clear when looking at the responses quoted here that many of the conditions that featured most regularly have a singular root cause: long-term stress. Many of the physical conditions experienced by these women are manifestations of a body and a brain that are overwhelmed: migraines, irritable bowel syndrome, specific and generalized anxiety disorders, chronic fatigue syndrome (CFS, also known as ME) and fibromyalgia are all reported by individuals and support services as anecdotally mentioned by autistic women. Liane Holliday Willey (2012) goes so far as to state that her gastrointestinal doctor believes that stress led to the loss of her gallbladder and removal of most of her sigmoid colon.

Autistic women are also particularly vulnerable to psychiatric disorders according to a population-based study of more than 1.3 million individuals (Martini *et al.*, 2022) which showed that 77 per cent of autistic women (compared with 66% of autistic men) would receive a diagnosis of at least one psychiatric condition and that 32 per cent of autistic women would be hospitalized (compared to 19% of autistic men). These figures were higher than those for non-autistic individuals.

These are the consequences of living in a world that is unknown, unpredictable and unsafe, both socially and physically. In treating and working with autistic women, we must take the autism into account when proposing treatment; it may be that the best 'cure' for some of these physical and mental conditions is in supporting a greater self-understanding for the individual, which will allow her to know her limitations and assert herself in making them known to others. I know for myself that it has been literally lifesaving for me to understand how limited my capacity is compared with others, and that regardless of how it appears, it is essential for me to limit my activities and put my own health above appearing 'normal'. I also have to ask those around me to do the same on my behalf when I am unable to due to my own urge to do everything. This process is also a painful one, as it means accepting limitations and 'inadequacy' (in my mind).

Autistic burnout

> I've asked doctors over and over why I am so exhausted, with no answers coming from the tests they did. It was a very frustrating experience. They acted like exhaustion was normal.

Until recently, the concept of 'burnout' was something reserved solely for the world of employment, being used to describe exhaustion as a result of overwhelming demands. 'Autistic burnout' appears to have developed through anecdotal accounts and social media, and the term has been recognized by autistic people as a useful way to describe their experiences of fatigue, mental distress and overwhelm in all areas of life. Periods of burnout are described as arising after particularly stressful events, or as existing almost constantly throughout life. Increased mental health issues, suicidal ideation and masking all contribute to autistic people's sense of feeling unable to cope with the huge effort required simply to exist, and can lead to autistic burnout. The topic has been entirely unresearched until recently and as yet has no established diagnostic basis, but early studies reveal themes of autistic burnout that many can resonate with.

Raymaker *et al.* (2020, p.140) suggest the following definition for autistic burnout:

> Autistic burnout is a syndrome conceptualized as resulting from chronic life stress and a mismatch of expectations and abilities without adequate supports. It is characterized by pervasive, long-term (typically 3+ months) exhaustion, loss of function, and reduced tolerance to stimulus.

Higgins *et al.* (2021, p.2365) suggest the following preliminary defined criteria which were derived following research and consultation with autistic adults:

> Autistic burnout is a severely debilitating condition with an onset preceded by fatigue from camouflaging or masking autistic traits, interpersonal interactions, an overload of cognitive input, a sensory environment unaccommodating to autistic sensitivities and/or other additional stressors or changes... The condition is not better explained by a psychiatric illness such as depression, psychosis, personality disorder, and trauma- and stressor-related disorders.

Autistic burnout often appears for the first time during adolescence (Mantzalas *et al.*, 2022). It can last for months or even years and tends to recur, resulting in autistic people struggling to maintain functional and meaningful lives. A difficulty in identifying one's own emotions and sensations – alexithymia – can contribute to autistic women not being aware of the early signs of burnout and therefore not being able to take steps to stop its progress to something more severe and life-limiting. The ability to manage the potential of burnout is directly related to the energy reserves of the person at any given time (Higgins *et al.*, 2021), and therefore failing to monitor and manage these energy levels due to alexithymia becomes a critical issue. The chronic exhaustion which follows can make it even more difficult to implement strategies for recovery.

> [...] Having all of your internal resources exhausted beyond measure and being left with no clean-up crew. (Raymaker *et al.*, 2020, p.136)

> Autistic burnout is when I no longer have the energy reserves to act neurotypical. (Higgins *et al.*, 2021, p.2360)

The experience of autistic burnout is widely considered to be poorly understood by others outside of the autistic community and often dismissed by professionals. The additional tendency for some autistic women to mask the visible presentations of their struggles can be a further trigger for autistic burnout as the cost of the camouflaging efforts required add to the already substantial burden of living in a non-autistic world, aggravating pre-existing stressors and leading to depression and suicidal ideation (Higgins *et al.*, 2021).

> I had my most intense period of autistic burnout before I realized I was autistic. It was at a time when I was working full-time hours in an open-plan office. The sensory bombardment I suffered every day was painful and draining. I knew I was struggling to connect with my co-workers, but despite my best attempts to fit in, I was being bullied and excluded. I'd also doubled my workload since starting the role, and even though I had explained this to senior managers, I was simply told that I had to get on with it, and my suggestions of prioritizing certain work were dismissed. One day I just couldn't get up. Everything felt like it was happening in slow motion. Words wouldn't come to me, and I felt physically exhausted. I had been coping and struggling on for so long that it felt like my brain had decided it needed to overrule me. Not knowing I was autistic meant that I was always comparing myself to the wrong people and pushing myself to be someone I wasn't. It was a terrifying time. I didn't know if my words would come back. I didn't have the energy to do anything. It wasn't depression, I wasn't sad or numb: I was just completely drained cognitively.
>
> It took me several weeks before my head began to clear enough to make some decisions. I ended up drastically changing my lifestyle in order to support my recovery. I moved to a new area and found a new part-time role in a lovely, small office. I found out later that after resigning, they had had to hire two people to cover all my work. The funny thing is that had the sensory environment been right, and the people around me understanding, I would have carried on doing all that work quite happily. I burnt myself out because I wasn't allowed to be who I am. Since realizing I'm autistic I plan my energy levels better. I work from home now, meaning my sensory environment is

> perfect and no one can ambush me with small talk. I still work too hard, but I balance that with working on projects that I love and that energizes me. When I burnt myself out there was no autistic joy in my life; now I make time to recover and do the things that spark my fascination. I will always be drained and exhausted by over-processing, but I hope to never go back to that time of utter emptiness ever again.

Due to the paucity of research and coherent definition of autistic burnout – as well as late diagnosis meaning that often adult autistic women only realize that they have experienced autistic burnout in hindsight following their autism diagnosis – recovery strategies are anecdotal and shared via autistic communities, often online through social media. Alone-time is an important feature of this recovery along with time spent on personal interests before a gradual return to daily activities and responsibilities (Higgins *et al.*, 2021; Neville, 2022).

> A week by the seaside has a truly a remarkable effect on me; not only because going away reduces the demands on me, but because the seaside is my favourite sensory environment to be in. I love the noise of the waves, the sight of the sea, the smell of salt; I love spinning and spinning on the beach. A week of restorative stimming, sensory pleasure, reduced demands, no socialising, and a change of scenery is the best thing I can do to prevent or treat my autistic burnout. (Garvey, 2023, p.228)

Alexithymia

> This often comes up for me in therapy, where my therapist will ask how I feel about something, or *where* I feel an emotion in my body, and I can't tell her. I've had this issue in therapy for years. I'm rarely able to identify how I'm feeling other than 'bad' or 'good'. I usually deal with the fall-out of my emotions rather than the emotions themselves. For example, I won't know I'm

> stressed until I scream at someone or throw something. I won't know I'm sad until my third day unable to get out of bed.

Alexithymia is a personality feature without a clear classification. It broadly relates to the difficulty in verbalizing emotions, which in turn relates to being unaware of the bodily sensations and feelings which correspond to these emotions. Also involved is a difficulty in being able to imagine what something might feel like for oneself and, as a result, challenges in imagining what things might feel like for other people and recognizing the visual signs of that. My own experience has always been that I have to carry out a feasibility study to determine what is the most likely cause of any physical sensation that I am feeling. If I have tightness in my chest, I have to think about what events have happened, or are soon to take place, that may explain anxiety, indigestion, heart attack, sugar crash or any other possibility. I am always completely exhausted by all people interaction, usually accompanied by excessive and odorous anxiety sweating, but I do not 'feel' anxious at all. When public speaking, my partner, Keith, would tell me that I looked like I was enjoying myself, but I had no sense of doing so or any other emotion. I have panic attacks at the thought of getting on a plane, but I have no conscious fear of flying. When asked how I feel, my typical response is 'I don't know', and even after considering the question logically for some time, I conclude that 'Nope, I really don't know'. The exclusions to this are physically overwhelming joy (always when outdoors in nature) and a deep and physically painful sense of loss (when thinking about people in my life).

> I often thought I 'went from 0 to 90' with my emotions. But when I actually examine those situations, I now recognise that I simply didn't notice that my emotions were climbing to 90. I might have felt an increased heart rate, or a tightening of my jaw, or a knot in my gut. I might have ignored those feelings, or been so focused on processing a conversation, trying to fit in socially, or trying to organise my thoughts, that I didn't give time to the emotional clues that were happening in my body. (Garvey, 2023, p.181)

> I had no understanding of what I felt as a young adult, which I think left me very vulnerable. I might occasionally, when exhausted, take time off from people and sit up into the small hours, crying, but I'm not sure I understood why. I certainly didn't understand I was autistic... In my 20s, a tutor told me I was like blotting paper, soaking up everyone else's emotions. When I had my first child and when she was born, I experienced something I had not before and to which I could not put a name. It was weeks, months later, I realized that what I had experienced, when I first set eyes on my baby girl, was joy.

Higher levels of alexithymia in autistic women rather than autism itself are connected to less accuracy in identifying emotions, and the difficulty in recognizing one's own emotions is related to being able to accurately read the facial expressions of others (Ola and Gullon-Scott, 2020). Alexithymia, therefore, can make it hard to establish close social relationships since the recognition, understanding and expression of emotions in both self and others are critical in knowing how to respond socially. There is no suggestion that there is a lack of emotion itself, simply a lack of visual or verbal emotional response.

> I feel like I've only got primary-colour emotions rather than a full rainbow complement, and I'm completely incapable of missing people, or feeling hungry until I'm actually starving!... It's extremely difficult to describe my feelings to others in anything other than an abstract way as I have synaesthesia too. If I'm unwell for example, I might just have an inner experience of electrical interference or the colour dark green, none of which sits on a GP's diagnostic checklist.

> I wonder often about alexithymia in terms of how other people misattribute language – facial expressions – body language in terms of emotion and/or pain, and feed those misattributions back to the person experiencing an emotion and/or pain. I know if I'm in pain, but my husband was the first person who

> understood what it looks like when I am in pain, based on how I express it. Similarly, as a child, my meltdowns were always read as anger and my shutdowns as sulking, so it took me until my 40s before I learned for myself what anger actually felt like, because I'd always been told that I was angry when I was in fact overwhelmed. I had to relearn what I'd known as a child but been taught otherwise.

For some, this can lead to a delay in emotional response, and these women have described how they feel and show nothing in the moment of witnessing their own or others' distress, but later collapse exhausted as the nature of what has occurred hits them. In terms of managing emotional situations, Dr Catriona Stewart OBE, autistic woman and founder of the Scottish Women's Autism Network, suggests (2022) that gender expectations for females mean that they are expected to be more emotionally driven rather than crisis managers or problem solvers, which is often what autistic females prioritize. She says: 'It's not that we don't have the emotions, it's more that we deal with them after the event'.

> The emotions thing I think is wrapped up with masking for me. My brain is cognizant of what has been said, for example. Say someone has had good news. I know it's good to feel happy for that person – which I do. I just have to remind my face to look that way. I am constantly managing my facial expression to ensure it's appropriate and as expected. However, if I'm concentrating or distracted or tired I don't manage to.

A connection between autism and alexithymia has been considered since the mid-1990s (Poquérusse *et al.*, 2018). While the link between the two is not entirely clear, it is suggested that higher proportions of autistic people experience it – 40 to 60 per cent (Griffin, Lombardo and Auyeung, 2016; Poquérusse *et al.*, 2018) – than within the general population – 10 per cent (Linden, Wen and Paulus, 1995) – but that despite a clear overlap, it is not a diagnostic feature of autism itself. More research is required for a fuller understanding of how they intersect, but an acceptance of the possibility of alexithymia can be helpful in knowing why there is either no reaction or a delayed one to a seemingly important emotional event. In my experience, autistic women often feel a great sense of shame about what has been perceived as 'coldness' in the face of the distress of others, even at times wondering if they are sociopaths. This knowledge of possible alexithymia as an explanation may in some way help to relieve this shame.

> I always thought I was fine at describing my emotions but after more research realize that I am not great at it at all. I have to logically work out what I am feeling, and it does not feel intuitive to me. I have been known to Google the differences between feeling angry or anxious (chemically they have very similar effects on the body, which I think confuses me). I have looked at feelings charts/wheels and they baffle me – I don't understand how people can know they are feeling such nuanced emotions.

> I'm currently trying to practise naming emotions as I feel the 'after-effects'. For example, if I start spiralling about something that's happened with a friend and try to think my way out of the problem, I practise saying to myself, 'I'm feeling anxious,' or 'This is anxiety'. This is extremely hard for me and it's not my natural inclination yet, but I do think it's a good exercise. Something about naming the emotion helps me realize it's temporary and I won't always feel like this.

Hypermobility/Ehlers–Danlos syndromes

Autism and hypermobility spectrum disorders (HSDs), which include Ehlers–Danlos syndrome (EDS), share a number of clinical features including sensory hypersensitivity, motor difficulties, mood disorders, epilepsy and proprioceptive impairment (Casanova *et al.*, 2020; Glans *et al.*, 2022). Typically, symptoms include increased range of joint movement (which can cause frequent dislocation), fragile skin that bruises or damages easily, digestive problems, dizziness and bladder control problems. Hypermobility disorders can be experienced mildly or be very debilitating. Joint hypermobility is fairly common and unless other symptoms are present wouldn't necessarily be an HSD or any cause for concern. HSDs, including EDS, are classed as hereditary connective tissue disorders, of which there are currently 14 types, 13 of which are considered rare and affecting extremely small numbers of people. The remaining subtype hypermobile EDS (HEDS) is strongly suggested to be a common condition accounting for 80 to 90 per cent of all EDS cases and is mostly diagnosed in women (Casanova *et al.*, 2020).

> [...] Hypermobility in several joints (identified by chiropracter as 4/9 on the Beighton Score). Posture stooped, joint instability, possibly also the link between hypermobility and blood circulation: blood can pool in lower part of body and result in a stress reaction on standing (this is from chiropracters: they think it might in part explain morning anxiety when I get up suddenly with the alarm clock).

One recent study (Glans *et al.*, 2022) suggests that autism and HSD are related conditions in adults, but that the high prevalence of attention deficit hyperactivity disorder (ADHD) in the study sample makes it difficult to generalize as to whether ADHD is the primary link here, or autism. More research is needed on individuals with only an autism diagnosis to verify this further. Other work (Casanova *et al.*, 2020) finds that autism and HSD occur within the same families and that 20 per cent of mothers with HSD have autistic children – a not significantly different rate than children born by autistic mothers.

One issue regarding the diagnosis of autism and co-morbid hypermobility is that these two conditions are dealt with and diagnosed clinically by entirely separate fields of medicine, which do not routinely overlap, leading to possible under-diagnosis of both. Pain may also remain untreated in autistic individuals due to communication differences; and a possible atypical perception of pain due to sensory differences means that it is important that any link between these conditions is known in order to anticipate possible pain management requirements (Baeza-Velasco *et al.*, 2018). Twenty per cent of children at one pain clinic presented with autism spectrum disorder (ASD) traits (Bursch *et al.*, 2004).

> I haven't officially been diagnosed with EDS, but it's come up a number of times with various doctors/chiropractors as a possibility. It all boils down to frequent injuries. Once, in my 20s, I went for a long walk and my knees became so painful I had to walk with a cane for two weeks. No doctor or MRI could find anything 'wrong' with my knees. In my early 30s I got pregnant, and my low back became so painful I couldn't shower or go to the bathroom by myself for weeks. I've gotten low-back flare-ups every few months. Thanks to a great physical therapist my flare-ups are way fewer and far between, but some activities I love like horseback riding and gardening are just no longer accessible to me because of this. The long and short of it is that very small, seemingly 'normal' and low-impact activities can sometimes trigger extreme pain.

> I have Ehlers–Danlos syndrome hypermobility type. It was diagnosed in my late 30s based on my bendy limbs. I sought diagnosis after a physiotherapist asked me if I knew I was hypermobile – I'd been having physiotherapists intermittently for more than a decade at that point. I had always had problems with my joints; my back and neck were particularly prone to causing me issues – I first put my back out when I was 14. I often sprained my ankles or hurt my wrists or elbows when putting my joints under strain, but it was only during my second pregnancy that the issues became intolerable. When my ligaments softened further due to pregnancy hormones, my hip joints destabilized to the point where I couldn't walk. I was diagnosed with pelvic girdle pain or symphysis pubis dysfunction (depending on which healthcare professional term they decided to use that day). My hips improved several months after giving birth, but they have

> never fully healed. I have to be careful to manage my weight and muscle strength around the joints or it reduces how far I can walk. I'm not supposed to run or do anything that puts strain on the joints. I have to be careful if I walk over a few miles or if I do anything that moves my legs at unusual angles.
>
> I always have to consider my limits: if I don't do enough exercise I'll lose muscle tone and put on weight, and that will strain my joints; if I do too much exercise that will put pressure on my loose ligaments and potentially damage the joints. It also means I'm at an increased risk of arthritis and general joint pain as I age. It's nice to be flexible but not nice enough to justify the pain that goes with it. When I was pregnant my husband compared me to one of those toys where you press a button underneath and the figure collapses. When your joints are too loose, that can be what it feels like – there's nothing to stop you falling to the ground in an untidy heap.

There is no specific treatment for HSD, but symptoms can be managed via physiotherapy, occupational therapy and also counselling to deal with feelings resulting from living with the condition. It may be advisable to avoid certain physical activities, wear protective clothing for other activities and increase lower impact exercise such as swimming or pilates which may help relieve symptoms.

> [...] Chiropracter for joint alignment: I should be doing exercises for core strength – joint stability but I'm not good at actually doing them!

> [...] I don't really, I live with chronic pain... I see a physical therapist once a month and try to keep on top of my exercises. I'm unable to do anything high intensity and it's not super fun to only do gentle movement like walking, yoga and physical therapy, but the risk far outweighs the reward, so I try to keep it simple to avoid injury.

Menstruation

Understanding before the onset of periods that they are a normal part of life and nothing to be concerned about reduces the surprise factor. Having a smaller social network may mean that some autistic girls do not have the peer support of those who have experienced their first period to normalize the experience. Practical considerations such as keeping clean, changing sanitary protection and avoiding mishaps are skills that may need to be taught and made part of a daily routine for young autistic women reaching puberty. Liane Holliday Willey (2012) describes her frequent 'accidents' with forgetting to change tampons, resulting in blood stains on furniture. Tracking menstrual cycles and developing an awareness of changing mental and physical symptoms may help autistic women to be prepared for the forthcoming period.

> I had to get my head around how she does everything literally, like I would say 'OK when you're finished with your pads you need to put them in the bin', so Hannah would walk through the house with them in her hand...they weren't wrapped up or anything... You have to go, 'OK, I need to think about how Hannah needs to hear this'. (Cridland *et al.*, 2014, p.1268)

In the group of participants that I questioned for this book, there were no significant differences in the age of starting menstruation than would be expected from the general population, and this is also seen in studies on this topic (Burke *et al.*, 2010).

> I was 12 when my periods started, and I hated it with a passion. Mum hadn't told me anything about them, and I didn't have other girls to tell me, although the school did a talk about it. During the talk I was pretty horrified at what I was hearing, and I think I prevented myself from taking it in. I remember they passed round a sanitary towel, and I refused to touch it. I think I concluded that 'No thank you, this stuff wasn't going to happen to me!'

> I didn't present as a typical girl, and it was difficult for me to identify with standard female roles or ideas of femininity... Puberty for me was the trenches. I had had extremely painful and heavy periods from the onset, which would cause me to vomit and have stomach upsets. Trying to manage this at school was traumatic, my family were unhelpful and unsupportive, my mental health deteriorated and I experienced depression for the first time. I hated being a girl so much that I starved myself so that my periods would stop. I then maintained a low body weight for most of my teens to avoid menstruation; I was diagnosed with anorexia nervosa, but it was more about not being ready for puberty rather than weight or body image. I purposefully put myself into hormonal stasis until I was emotionally ready to manage my adult female body.

Higher rates of premenstrual syndrome (PMS) and dysmenorrhoea have been seen in autistic women compared to neurotypical women (Hamilton *et al.*, 2011). Obaydi and Puri (2008) found that 92 per cent of autistic women with intellectual disabilities experienced PMS in their study compared to 11 per cent of the non-autistic control group. There is some suggestion too that autistic people may experience a higher level of hormone fluctuation than neurotypical peers (Obaydi and Puri, 2008). Ingudomnukul *et al.* (2007) also found that significantly more autistic women experienced irregular menstrual cycles, dysmenorrhoea and polycystic ovary syndrome (PCOS), and made connections with elevated testosterone levels in autistic individuals. They found that almost twice as many autistic women experienced PMS than non-autistic controls. Another study (Pohl *et al.*, 2014) found that autistic women showed higher frequencies of epilepsy, PCOS, atypical menstruation and severe acne than the control group. PCOS was mentioned by a number of the women I questioned as being something that they had been diagnosed with, and this does appear to be a relatively common feature for autistic women. The exact frequency cannot be estimated as it is likely that there are a significant number of women who have undiagnosed PCOS.

In Obaydi and Puri's (2008) study of autistic women with intellectual disabilities, the autistic group were seen to present increased irritability, anger, social withdrawal and impaired performance during the premenstrual phase. Another study showed an increase in self-injurious behaviours and mood dysregulation (Lee, 2004). Some of these impacts may be connected to a difficulty in communicating discomfort and pain or in understanding what is happening. Asking for support and self-soothing may also be more difficult for those with intellectual disabilities and limited verbal communication.

In a more recent study by Steward *et al.* (2018), autistic participants reported that autism-related challenges made life more difficult to manage during menstruation, which reflect the earlier research.

> [...] Hates her period (she is hyper-aware of it and finds it hard to focus on other things). (Parent)

Feeling more sensitive to smell, touch and other stimuli, when accompanied by menstrual pain, can lead to an inability to focus on anything other than the sensory experience. Executive functioning and general life management are reported to worsen during this time.

Polycystic ovary syndrome (PCOS)

It may be a coincidence or evidence of serendipity that at the same time I was working on writing this section, I was reading *Travels with Charley* by John Steinbeck (1962) in which he says: 'in our time a beard is the one thing a woman cannot do better than a man' (p.32). I beg to differ, Mr Steinbeck, as some of us may well have whooped you on that one too. Given that I have PCOS, and thanks to the enhanced beard-growing quality that this brings, I own more pairs of tweezers than any single person should – a pair in each room in the house, a pair in each bag and a pair in the car – in order to keep my magnificent beard at bay. I suppose it's best that I keep it in check to allow gentlemen like Mr Steinbeck to continue to believe that they have at least one thing to offer. As we shall see, PCOS is a collection of seemly disparate symptoms all of which can add up to considerable discomfort and problems. For me, irregular periods, difficulty managing carbohydrates (insulin resistance), easy weight gain and that eternal beard have all been a constant bane of my life. And then we find out that it all might be connected to autism...

PCOS is caused by elevated levels of testosterone, which causes fluid-filled sacs in the ovaries and results in infertility, irregular menstruation, insulin resistance and excess bodily hair. Elevated levels of prenatal testosterone have been suggested as a factor in the development of autism, and thus researchers have investigated the idea that women with PCOS could have elevated autistic traits. Their findings suggest that women with PCOS have a greater chance of having an autistic child compared to a woman without PCOS. They also found out that autistic women are more likely to have PCOS and that women with PCOS were more likely to be autistic, as expected (Cherskov *et al.*, 2018). Daughters of women with PCOS also scored more highly on autistic traits, but not their sons (Kosidou *et al.*, 2016).

> [...] Diagnosed when I was 19 years old. I was told that I was infertile and my chances of conceiving naturally were very slim. However, I fell pregnant with twins when I was 20. I also had an ectopic pregnancy when I was 29 whilst using the Mirena coil. The doctors said that both the twins and ectopic pregnancy were likely caused due to my PCOS. Problems with sugar – make me crash and my eyes go funny (very heavy and like I can't focus properly). I try to eat a lower carb/sugar diet but struggle as I love carbs and sweet things! I also seem to be much hairier than other women: spiky chin hairs since I was in my 20s that I have to pluck regularly, and other body hair grows back very quickly!

> I have PCOS: I was a tomboy as a child, preferred to play with the boys; as a young adult, developed hirsuitism, especially face, and worsening as I get older. I need to watch my blood sugar: sugary

> things cause a rebound effect, so I generally avoid... In those days, i.e. when I was young, PCOS wasn't widely recognized, and while I did go to my GP in my early 20s, she couldn't offer me any route to a diagnosis or any treatment. It was only some years later, I think it was a hairdresser told me, she thought I had it and I should go to see a herbalist for help. So I did.

Menopause

> My menopause experience was entirely positive. I suffered 40 years of severe premenstrual tension: horrible period pains that required regular pain relief for the first two days of my periods and left me feeling sick. The realization at the age of 53 that my periods had stopped for good was freeing and positive. What were a few hot flushes and a bit of vaginal atrophy in comparison to the preceding 40 years? Nothing to worry about at all.

The majority of adult women who contact me regarding undertaking an assessment for autism are in their 40s to 60s, and most cite a sense of being unable or unwilling to keep up the pretence of trying to be 'normal' any more, which has come upon them in recent years. A feeling that they just can't be bothered to continue doing things which have little meaning to them, and which have led to illness and exhaustion – combined with their continued experience that life is harder for them than for their peers – brings them to a crisis point. This revelation and decision to let the mask drop seem to come at a time of life when the hormonal changes defined as menopausal have become part of the picture. Little is known about the effect of perimenopause on autistic women, with one of the earliest mentions coming from autistic author Cynthia Kim in her wonderful book *Nerdy, Shy and Socially Inappropriate* (2014) where she wondered whether menopause would affect her differently than her neurotypical peers.

Christine Jenkins, autistic advocate and Community Research Associate at Carleton University in Canada, is working with a

Canadian/UK research team on the Bridging the Silos project on autistic menopause, which is the first large-scale study of women's experiences and seeks to bridge the gaps between different menopausal perspectives from gynaecologists, psychologists and autistic women, bringing them together to share knowledge and learn from each other. The first part of the project, which involved focus groups and asking menopausal women to submit creative expressions of their experiences, can be found at the website[1] and a wider survey of autistic women's experiences is taking place in 2023, with findings expected to published on its completion.

Some qualitative studies are beginning to shed some light on this experience (Karavidas and de Visser, 2022; Moselely, Druce and Turner-Cobb, 2021). The first of these studies also found that a proportion of the participants had sought autism diagnosis as a result of the heightened difficulties that resulted from their menopausal experience, which corroborates my own professional experience.

> I didn't even suspect that I was autistic until my perimenopausal symptoms became a significant problem. I would say that the perimenopause 'outed' my autism, that the level of masking need to function at work became unmanageable.

> Being undiagnosed (autistic) masked my early perimenopause symptoms, such as night sweats, anxiety and depression, and they were continually diagnosed as mental health disorders... I was diagnosed autistic in 2021, a month after I realized I was six years into my perimenopause and still battling with my GP to agree with me, so it's impossible to know what symptoms were autistic traits/trauma and what was perimenopause.

Just to make things worse, menopause tends to arrive at a time in life where other colossal changes are also occurring. The death of parents and older relatives, children leaving home, downsizing and general physical limitations of ageing can all prove to be

1 www.autisticmenopause.com

overwhelming in addition to menopausal symptoms, and it is important to be aware of this and find appropriate support. As autistic people, we don't 'do' change well at the best of times, but this altered mental state can certainly make things worse, and, as ever, knowing that you are not weak/broken/failing can be hugely valuable.

> When I hit 50, everything 'fell apart'. I was in a new job, new tasks, new team, heavy workload; I'd not slept a full night in a year, had days when my head felt completely empty, and was bleeding heavily, irregularly, and sometimes for three to six weeks without a break... And I didn't realize I was autistic.

Other autistic women have reported that they failed to identify the cause of menopausal changes which brought new physiological and physical discomfort (Karavidas and de Visser, 2022) as being distinct from those experienced throughout their lives – this being a default state for autistic women. I relate to this strongly myself having slowly realized that I have frequently become suddenly hot for years but had just assumed that other people were feeling the same!

> I was raising two teenage girls as a single parent, working hard, physically running around all over the place, stressed about money and that I had a special educational needs child, etc.... So, my menopause was conducted to that background noise! I started the menopause some time before realizing I was autistic myself, so it's hard to know what was menopausal, what were increased stress reactions.

> I started to cry a lot in my mid-40s, but it took a further seven years to realize that this was just the beginning of perimenopause.

> I lost my confidence and could feel myself disappearing. My sleep and dreams became bizarre and disturbed; I was sad, hopeless, nostalgic and tearful. Pre-existing migraines and

> tinnitus have become worse. All of the above are classic symptoms of menopause, but because my typical autistic experience has always been fraught with discomfort, anxiety and strange physical sensations, I didn't put it all together.

Once perimenopause had been identified as the cause of these new symptoms, a whole raft of unwanted physical experiences ensued:

> The worst thing for me was the heat/hot flushes and that I broke out in acne rosaceae, which never goes away once you start it. I also started getting rheumatism in my late 40s, fingers mostly then.

> Low energy, less capacity, endometriosis worsened, joint pain, hair loss, headaches, hot flashes and night sweats. Vaginal atrophy, which required treatment; it was very difficult physically.

> Awful night sweats, vaginal dryness, menstrual migraines.

> Nights sweats, poor sleep, the beginnings of brain fog, loss of confidence.

Anxiety and depression, which are already present, worsen for many, and emotions appear heightened and more reactive to unexpected events. For me, this has marked the end of more than a decade of public speaking/training work as the panic attacks I suddenly started experiencing both on stage and on public transport have made it too uncomfortable for me to continue to travel and present.

> Anxiety and depression increased, the insomnia was brutal, my mood was low most of the time, and I lost interest in, and the enjoyment of, a lot of things.

> Anger was amplified, I felt like I was in 'Hulk Smash' mode for a long time, especially whilst driving or at work.

> My anxiety went through the roof... I was having palpitations, awake for hours worrying about the 'smallest' things.

> I am generally quite kind, but I found this more difficult; it upsets me at times how I struggled to give a shit about things!

Some reported that they were less tolerant or capable of social interaction and had increased difficulties with both verbal and non-verbal communication and in tolerating previous manageable changes to plans.

> [...] Totally retreated into my shell, didn't want to see people or leave the house... Found conversations harder, couldn't mask, didn't know how to be around people and not mask.

> Increases in anxiety levels, tiredness meaning my capacity to do more than the basics, and brain fog all meant my tolerance for change was almost nil. Once I'd planned something any changes would leave me in tears/bed.

Sensory experiences can also be heightened, making functioning difficult.

> [...] All increased, especially sensitivity to smells, noises and that feel of fabrics on my skin.

> Clothing feels 'heavy', bedsheets feel rough, sanitary pads/tampons are uncomfortable. Walking/moving with clothes on feels hard some days.

> My capacity to cope with sensory overload decreased, along with my capacity to cope with everything else, and things I'd previously coped with became unmanageable/things I actively avoided, e.g. the workplace, cafés and restaurants.

In terms of obtaining medical support for menopausal symptoms, some autistic women found a lack of understanding from professionals (Moseley, Druce and Turner-Cobb, 2020) of both their autistic experience and their additional, sometimes atypical, menopausal experience. It can also be difficult for autistic women to manage the requirements of treatment and medication, even if it is forthcoming. For those who have been able to access treatment, some have found it beneficial.

> I don't know if I am perimenopausal because my health is so poor anyway that it's difficult to know what is causing what symptoms day to day (given my age I probably am), but I do know that HRT [hormone replacement therapy] has helped with lifelong mental health symptoms that I think are partially associated with autism. HRT has reduced what I call 'autistic inertia', a.k.a. the ability to start a task that really needs doing, but the effort required to get started is frequently too large to overcome.

> I had a very early menopause (40), and I should have been referred to an early menopause clinic, but it was all blamed on mental health and I was probably three years in before I realized that it was perimenopause. I have recently had a new GP, and they have been helpful. I have been prescribed vaginal oestrogen and that has relieved some of my symptoms.

> I really struggled to order HRT meds from the GP and collect them from the chemist in time, just too hard / another thing to do when I was overwhelmed and exhausted.

> I was on oestrogen gel and the performance of rubbing it in and being sticky was really difficult. I hate being sticky! It took me around three months to get anywhere near regular to using it.

As has often been the case, autistic women become 'experts' in themselves and the medical conditions that affect them. Participants in the same study (Moseley *et al.*, 2020) also expressed a difficulty in determining what was 'normal' for them to expect, given that general information on menopause is limited and that this may not entirely apply to them anyway. Autistic people with limited communication abilities may especially struggle to make their discomfort known within this context of limited information and understanding from professionals.

> When I did go [to the GP], I was well-informed (Balance Menopause website, Dr Louise Newson), and my GP readily agreed to prescribing HRT.

> By the time I was finally given HRT, I could barely walk up the stairs as every muscle and bone in my body ached. I couldn't focus on conversations with anyone as I just couldn't remember any words... I was heavily medicated with antidepressants, yet still no one was taking me seriously. I do believe that my masking abilities covered up the extent of my struggle.

> HRT is the only thing that helped initially. And then, about ten months after I started on the HRT, as my strength started to return more noticeably, I started cutting out salt and refined sugar from my diet, which has helped a lot with energy levels and water retention.

Positive aspects of menopause reported by participants (Moseley *et al.*, 2020) included the joy of the cessation of periods, a freedom from social and sexual pressures of being female - an increased invisibility brought about by ageing and being seen as less desirable - and making better choices for themselves in terms of self-care.

The realization of perimenopause as an explanation has been as powerful as the realization of autism as an explanation for myself and other autistic women. I wasn't mad, I wasn't broken, I wasn't mentally ill; my hormones were just erratically changing and causing havoc with my mind and body. What a relief! Since this discovery, things have vastly improved for me. On the positive side, after a lifetime of trying to appease people, hide all of who I am and apologize for my existence, I appear to have lost the ability to give a f**k and have become shockingly assertive. What liberation. My anger has a voice for the first time in its life, and it's quite a loud one. Long live the demise of oestrogen! It seems that I am not alone:

> It [perimenopause] has 'outed' my autism, which has been such a good experience (if difficult) as now my life makes sense, I feel less of a failure, and I am beginning to make different choices for myself.

> I just don't tolerate my own boundaries being compromised in the same way. 'Jog on', 'your problem, not mine' and other phrases spring to mind much more readily...and I act on them in a way I wouldn't have had the confidence to before.

> I am through perimenopause now, but I feel like a badass for surviving it, I am no longer passive or a pushover, and I no longer feel that I have to 'please' others.

> I quite like being an 'elder'; I hate the weight gain and reduced energy, but I like no longer caring much what people think of me and feeling I can dispense wisdom and advice (even when not asked for it).

> Generally, people start leaving you alone in life when you turn 40! People stopped asking me when I was going to have children! Aside from that, I feel my life has gone from one traumatic event/period of time to another, so I am very much looking forward to being the other side of the menopause and (hopefully) having some kind of regularity to my life.

Depression

Depression was mentioned by around 50 per cent of the women questioned, and from my experience I would suggest that this figure is likely to be even higher across this population. The experience of feeling different, excluded and living in an unjust world, yet having no means to fix things, is so common to autistic people that many perhaps do not even relate to the term 'depression' – it's just 'life'. Many autistic women I have worked with described themselves as having been 'depressed forever' and felt that their low mood was simply a consequence of their limited social acceptance and daily challenges; they were unable to differentiate their depression from their autism. Problems with identifying emotional responses (alexithymia) from physical sensations can form part of this difficulty as they may not actually know how they are feeling and/or be able to articulate that into words. I also wonder (partly from my own perspective) whether having lived with a constant sense of low mood and stress for most of one's life results in someone not actually knowing what 'okay' feels like.

> [...] Depression since mid-teens. I feel it has limited my efforts to improve my situation [...] It's difficult to separate the impact of depression from that of Asperger's – I think the two have combined to isolate me for decades.

> I believe my depression is often triggered by an increase in anxiety and may be an effort to slow down and tone down the feelings of anxiety to the point that I think I no longer care about my well-being. I also frequently perseverate or fixate on issues that are bothering me in an effort to try to understand and resolve disturbances. However, often, this tendency and inability to stop thinking about issues has probably worsened my depression.

> I guess I have never lost hope that things will improve, however difficult, which I know is different to the classical description of depression. I feel like my depression is different to how other NT [neurotypical] people describe it.

Some women found that medication helped to lift their mood, but others had learned strategies to cope with this intrinsic part of their lives. They were stoic and aware in their responses about how to get themselves through it. Confidence in professional help was low, with most feeling that they were not understood by mental health professionals, whose knowledge of autism was perceived to be basic or non-existent. The women who had sought professional help tended to be those who had reached a very serious level of depression and saw it as a last resort.

> Learning to recognize when I am depressed is important, as it is insidious and can creep up unnoticed over a period of weeks or months. Once I notice I am depressed, sometimes it helps just to throw in the towel and 'nurse' myself for a couple of days by resting/eating as much as I feel like and having a break from normal activities, before coming up with a plan of action and getting back to a pattern of healthy activity and diet (although gently!).

> I need not to be nagged, not to have too much noise, not to be told that I have nothing to be depressed about and I should pull myself together. I actually tend to avoid people because often their reactions are unhelpful. I know how to get myself through it and would rather do it alone.

Anxiety

Anxiety is widely recognized as being a normal part of life for many people on the autism spectrum. We have seen previously that autistic women are in particular danger of being diagnosed with a mental health condition *instead* of an ASD (rather than *as well as*), so we may conclude they are more likely to present the symptoms of anxiety than autistic males. Anxiety was mentioned specifically by around 50 per cent of the women I questioned and is featured in most books written by and about autistic women (Holliday Willey, 2001; Lawson, 2000; Nichols *et al.*, 2009).

> The anxiety is an everyday, chronic problem that is greatly worsened under stressful conditions, often at work or in tense social situations. Since I tend to deteriorate under pressure (or have a meltdown more or less), I now also fear or have anxiety about not being able to handle future situations.

> It makes it difficult to plan things because sometimes I feel like doing something when I arrange it, but then on the day I can't face it. I let people down a lot and cancel things a lot.

> Anxiety can be crippling and all-consuming if someone makes things harder for me by failing to do something or lying. I don't feel depression as such, but I can get very down, again, when people make it tough for me.

Autistic women feel anxious because they live in a world that is endlessly confusing, illogical and frustrating, and full of inconsistencies and alterations to the status quo. This is perhaps exacerbated by the gender expectations placed on them, which they feel unable to meet. The result of all of this is sometimes avoidance of certain situations as well as a general sense of worry that can be triggered at any moment. The following are some of the circumstances that the autistic women found particularly stressful.

> I have to avoid situations that often contribute to my anxiety. I particularly get anxious when I am alone in crowds or in crowded situations or when I have to negotiate difficult social situations. I generally need some guidance, coaching or feedback to help me deal with and interpret these situations as a lot of my anxiety results from my inability to process information in real time.

> [...] Meeting someone I know but not that well suddenly on a bus, [at] a bus stop, in a café, etc. I find it very stressful trying to think what to say. I'd rather speak to someone I don't know at all.

Self-harm

> [...] Snapping rubber bands, cutting, punching walls, punching myself. Sometimes fasting 'til I can feel hunger pains and the empty growling sensation, sometimes eating until I feel painfully full because 'satisfied' isn't enough.

People self-harm in different ways and for different reasons. Sensory soothers and repetitive movements include finger- and skin-picking, scratching, rubbing and plucking hairs, which can be seen as harmful but may perform a positive function at the same time. How an individual chooses to frame these behaviours is personal, but perhaps the line between a sensory comfort and self-harm is a blurred one. Mothers of autistic girls report self-harm as being of particular concern (Stewart, 2012). My understanding is that girls and autistic women self-harm as a means of feeling something real (pain) in times of overwhelming emotion. Liane Holliday Willey (2012) describes her own 'scraping' as a means to reconnect with herself but cautions that others will assume that you are trying to hurt yourself rather than trying to (in some way) heal yourself.

As a teenager, I cut myself, a lot, although deliberately not to the degree that would require outside intervention and, therefore, unwanted attention. My weapon of choice was a safety pin. I would rub the open end over the skin on my hands and arms repeatedly until it bled and then continue to do so. I also etched boys' names and initials into my hands. I can still see faint scars now 40 years later. At the time I had no idea why I did it. I knew nothing about autism. I knew that I felt overwhelming physical sensations that welled up inside my body like a volcano with no vent, no outlet for release. I couldn't attach any words to these sensations and, put simply, I didn't know what to do with them. I couldn't speak about them as I had no words for them. This is now known to be alexithymia. Breaking my skin and channelling the feelings into physical pain somehow diverted my attention into something solid and tangible and made them dissipate. There was a sense of relief and calm.

Meditation, self-awareness and, certainly, a diagnosis of autism can all help girls and women to understand why they feel the way they do and raise awareness of how to manage it safely without causing physical harm. Telling a woman to stop self-harming without supporting her reasons for doing so is unlikely to be successful and more likely to make her feel like a failure for being 'found out' as not coping.

Alcohol and drug use

For others, alcohol and drugs may fulfil a similar function by blocking out emotional confusion and the feeling of being overwhelmed. Research into substance misuse in those on the autism spectrum is virtually non-existent. I co-wrote a book on the subject (Tinsley and Hendrickx, 2008), which presented evidence to suggest that social anxiety and alcoholism may be connected. Sixty-five per cent of individuals entering alcohol treatment centres have a diagnosis of social anxiety disorder. One study by van Wijnjgaarden-Cremers and van der Gaag (2015) suggested that there may be a link between autism and addiction and considers that there may be common factors which predispose autistic people to addiction. Historian Gilman Ostrander theorizes that alcoholism is a condition for individualists and loners who sense early on in their lives that they are alone in the world (cited in Goodwin, 1988).

The responses of the women I spoke to represent a wide range when it came to their consumption of legal and illegal substances. For some the idea of drinking was pointless, expensive and led to unwanted feelings of lack of control. 'Social drinking' was a bizarre concept to them and one which they could never relate to, further separating them from their peers, particularly in teens and early adulthood when drinking alcohol is core to social interaction.

For others, alcohol and drugs enabled social interaction by increasing tolerance of people and loud, otherwise overwhelming sensory environments. This was my experience as a teenager, and were it not for me becoming pregnant while drunk as a teenager – which halted my career as a burgeoning alcoholic drinking half a bottle of gin every afternoon at the age of 17 years – I strongly suspect that I would have got myself into serious trouble with my drinking.

> People were still smoking in offices and shared them around, and I did it to fit in... Cigarettes helped as they were an excuse to go and stand outside for ten minutes, or longer, every hour or so and have quiet, one-to-one conversations; they still help as a way of breaking up periods of activity.

> Smoking was also a way of making connections at work in a way that felt manageable... It created an opportunity to build superficial but useful networks across large organizations with people I wouldn't normally have contact with, and it meant I almost always knew someone when I walked into an event or meeting.

> I have used alcohol and stimulants to ease my anxiety when socializing, especially as a young person. I don't feel that I would have required these substances as much if I was not autistic.

> [...] Allow me to become a social butterfly – after a few drinks I could say pretty much whatever I thought.

> Using alcohol for the first time took away all my social fears and anxieties. I didn't know I was autistic and couldn't understand the difficulties I was having with my self-image and self-esteem at that time. Alcohol seemed a very easy and useful way to integrate myself into groups and feel good about myself whilst doing so.

> When I am drunk I don't care as much whether people secretly don't want to talk to me. Normally I am constantly aware of the possibility that I am not acting appropriately, and I stress out about it. Being drunk enables me to be someone else, superficially closer to the way that other people are. (Tinsley and Hendrickx, 2008, p.34)

> I am less afraid of novel things when drunk, which is why I am quite happy to talk to strangers and go to new places without having someone familiar with me. (Tinsley and Hendrickx, 2008, p.60)

> I often drink on my own before going out, so that I am confident when I arrive rather than being anxious at first. Then I drink more when I am out. (Tinsley and Hendrickx, 2008, p.60)

> I think I used to get high as a way of coping socially although didn't know that at the time because everyone else was doing it. I loved how everyone else was weird on drugs (like they had stepped into my world!) but found myself struggling to socialize without a drink.

> I think it's [substance use] given me the confidence to do things and be a kind of self-actualized version of myself. It's funny that most people associate negative things with drinking, but for me it's just allowed me to switch off the inhibitions and constant self-monitoring in real time.

For some of this group, the decreased inhibitions created by the substance combined with an autistic challenge of failing to read hidden agendas led to sexual assault, vulnerability to predatory behaviour from others and risk-taking. For others, this led to addiction.

> Drinking has given me short-term problems, such as feeling sick and having hangovers. I also tend to injure myself whilst drunk because I think it is a good idea to climb over fences rather than use gates, etc. (Tinsley and Hendrickx, 2008, p.77)

> I think the most detrimental effect has been the hundreds of idiots I've got off with in an attempt to find actual love; this has certainly put me in some dangerous situations that wouldn't have happened when sober. I remember going back to a guy's

> house because he seemed nice and I thought he might like me, but actually when I refused to sleep with him he was really verbally abusive, and I was actually terrified he'd rape me.

> I did some very dangerous things in my teens and early 20s – above and beyond what would be seen as 'normal'... I attempted to fly out of a bedroom window, walked on broken glass, slept with various men (not because I wanted to, but because I felt that I owed them...weirdly), and became very financially generous, with no concept of tomorrow. It was like being on a spiral of self-harm really, looking at these comments now.

> Substance use has had a hugely negative impact on my life, as I was rarely ever able to moderate my use, as a result leaving me regularly feeling unwell, with social consequences, and even more anxiety the following day... When eventually I was drinking to get drunk every single day, I realized that I could not stop. It took me to a very lonely, desperate place before I came into recovery (three years clean and sober).

> I could, and often would, take risks and put myself in danger. It made me vulnerable. I had people over the years take advantage of me whilst I was intoxicated.

> Drinking has always caused me to be more vulnerable socially, make poor choices and take risks that I would not take otherwise. I have started relationships during periods of drinking that were unhealthy for me and abusive. I have also been sexually assaulted when drunk.

One woman commented that drugs did not always have the same effect on her as they did for others.

> I noticed that substances like MDMA did not make me 'high' in the same way as allistic [non-autistic] people. I was not more social on these substances but insular and disconnected; they

> did increase my enjoyment of sensory stimuli such as music or images though. At a festival, I took MDMA with a group of friends; they all went dancing for the night, but I found the film tent and sat on my own watching Stanley Kubrick movies until the morning. It was wonderful!

Suicidal ideation

It has been suggested that autistic individuals may have suicidal thoughts and make plans for ending their own lives with greater frequency than would be expected in the general population (Cassidy *et al.*, 2014). This study found that 66 per cent of autistic adults had had thoughts about ending their lives. Autistic women without intellectual disability have a higher risk of suicidal behaviours than autistic males (Hirvikoski *et al.*, 2020). Those who camouflage are also said to be at greater risk of experiencing 'thwarted belongingness and lifetime suicidality' (Cassidy *et al.*, 2020, p.3638). The masking of autistic traits in social situations – and subsequent failure to successfully fit in – can lead to these feelings. This is something I wrote in Philip Wylie's book *Very Late Diagnosis of Asperger Syndrome* (2014) on the subject:

> My Aspie opinion of suicidal thinking is...maybe just a non-emotional, logical analysis of the situation: suicide is genuinely one of the potential options. I think neurotypical people can find suicidal thinking very shocking...whereas for some of us it's almost part of everyday life. (Hendrickx, in Wylie 2014, p.111)

Other women shared their recollections and thoughts about this topic. What comes across is pragmatism about the issue and the proposed solution. I wonder whether there is a difference in the emotions and thought processes involved in suicidal ideation for autistic people in comparison to neurotypical (NT) people. This is an as-yet unstudied area.

> I remember deciding that I would kill myself if I wasn't happier

> by the time I was 25 but had no specific measures for that happiness nor any specific plan in mind. I have occasionally considered suicide over the years, but I wouldn't say I have ever actually been suicidal. When I have thought about it, it has taken the form more of how I would organize things so as to minimize the trauma for others – write a letter to the police notifying them so that my body can be found by them rather than an acquaintance.

One woman articulated very clearly her conclusions about her own suicidal ideation and how this could apply to other autistic people. She also beautifully advises how this could be avoided for future generations.

> I do believe that we (autistic individuals such as myself) are very susceptible to suicidal thinking for multiple reasons that include: chronically high levels of anxiety, tendency to fixate on or get stuck on negative disturbing thoughts, low self-worth, inability to have significant or intimate relationships with others, replaying over and over again negative statements that others have said to us, feeling unable to be understood, lack [of] a solid self-identity, difficulty with expressing self to others, feelings of great isolation, feeling that you are or may be a burden to others, feeling unable to contribute to society or the greater good, etc... I do believe that the most important thing that someone else can do for a struggling autistic individual is to affirm their self-worth, recognize and validate their struggles and affirm the things that they do that are greatly valued by others. The worst thing to do for an autistic individual, or any struggling individual for that matter, is to not believe them or to deny the validity of their struggles. My greatest and deepest hurt is that doctors, family members and important others did not believe me in my struggles, particularly when I was younger, before my diagnosis at the age of 35 years. This has been the strongest impetus for my feelings of unworthiness and suicidal thoughts.

In the black-and-white cognitive processing world of autism, where multiple alternative strategies can be difficult to generate, suicide may be one of the few options that the person has found. Cognitive behavioural approaches that assist in perspective shifting and broadening may be helpful in supporting autistic women to come up with a greater number of options and assess their suitability. An autism-specific approach is required: that is, one that recognizes both the experience and the cognitive-processing style of an autistic person rather than generic, emotion-based therapeutic intervention.

> I've been in and out of cognitive behaviour therapy for 40 years and while it has helped me deal with many issues, I have yet to find the key that will lock stress out of my life. (Holliday Willey, 2012, p.63)

So, after that less than cheery run-down of all the potential ailments and challenges that may befall us, let's finish this journey with thoughts and possibilities for living well in this strange world that autistic females find themselves in.

Chapter 14

LIVING WELL IN A NON-AUTISTIC WORLD

'So, what now?' is a commonly asked question from autistic women and parents of autistic girls after the confirmation of diagnosis. Sadly, the answer is no quick fix. What autistic females need to do is to work out how to live well in a non-autistic world. Simple, eh?!

The best and most simple way of thinking about the impact of being autistic in a non-autistic world has already been mentioned by Jess in Chapter 12 on eating, and it is autism author, lecturer and simply marvellous bloke, Dr Luke Beardon's equation:

Autism + Environment = Outcome

What this tells us is that it is the environment that changes the outcome rather than autism, since the autistic profile of a person largely remains the same. 'Environment' in this context can mean anything at all that has an impact on the person and requires a response: rain, people, tiredness, an itchy jumper, a late train, the wrong sort of apple, a surprise, a facial expression, a joke, a party – you name it, it counts. What this equation offers is the opportunity to try to identify the factors which have caused the outcome – either negatively or positively – and find ways to either avoid them or incorporate more of them into your life.

A useful and tangible way to think about this is by using 'spoon theory', a concept developed in 2003 by Christine Miserandino as a way to manage her lupus. Christine used the idea of 'spoons' as units of energy and how she had to manage her availability of these spoons to carry out everyday tasks while in chronic pain. This idea can be useful for autistic people in terms of balancing obligations with physical and mental capacity to maintain wellness and also predict possible times where there may be a spoon deficit and find strategies to deal with this. It can be used too as a way of thinking about how spoon supply can be replenished and what activities or situations might enable this. For some it may be sleeping, for others exercise, interests, music and so on. It's all individual. For example, if I wake up in the morning and think about how I'm feeling: Did I sleep well? How much energy do I have? Let's say I think I have seven spoons to spend. I then may think about the day ahead; it may include shopping (two spoons), making a phone call (one spoon), working on the laptop (three spoons), picking up the kids from school (two spoons). This makes a total of eight spoons, and I haven't got to making dinner, playing with the kids, talking to my partner or tidying the house. This would be a negative spoon day.

So, I can either lay in bed and get super anxious about this or I can think about how I might manage my spoon count differently. I can get something out of the freezer for dinner, thereby avoiding going shopping (+ two spoons); I can put off making the phone call (+ one spoon); I can go for a run instead of going shopping (+ two spoons). Already, the day is looking better, and we are back in the black spoonwise. It's a basic example, but hopefully you get the point. As a parent or carer you can do the same with or for your children. Get them involved in identifying spoon counts for certain activities and also selecting spoon replenishment activities. This can help with emotional regulation and feeling more in control of situations and their outcomes. As a carer you will know what really causes stresses for your girls, and you will know what they need in those times. Drawing charts of spoons can make this idea really visual and concrete. And it doesn't have to be spoons – it can be manga characters, horses, Sherlock Holmes or balls of wool.

It's all about identifying and predicting energy credits and debits. I use the word 'framework' to explain how autism can be used as the baseline for identifying and understanding these stressors and sources of joy. Obviously, it can be limiting and impractical to try to avoid everything that is difficult and/or spend all of your days knitting when the dog needs taking for a walk. It is all about finding the small things that make the biggest differences. For example, in my former life as an on-the-road trainer and conference speaker, I spent numerous days in hotels, strange towns and training conference venues, in all of which I needed to eat. Now, I love food and can eat most things, but I am extremely sensitive to sugar/carbs particularly when in situations of high stress/adrenaline/cortisol (I don't have the space or skills to go into this in this book, but please check out links between sugar/carbs and anxiety, and then put down the Doritos). I also have polycystic ovary syndrome (PCOS), resulting in insulin resistance and sugary foods causing an immediate crash, which is not much help when you have to go back to deliver training after lunch. I found delivering training completely exhausting and had zero resources for chatting to people in the breaks, queuing for lunch and having to make decisions about which, if any, of the foods on offer would keep me going throughout the rest of the day. If lunch was not on offer, I would need to venture out into an unknown town in my break to source suitable foods (more people, more decisions, more anxiety). That was all too much for an overloaded me to handle (no spoons).

So, my simple solution was to find foods that managed my blood sugar, didn't need a fridge as my hotel room never had one (I'm a Travelodge kind of gal), could be made with a kettle and carried in a Tupperware, and eaten with my trusty titanium Spork. I give you sardine and couscous. By taking my own food I also avoided all people interactions, having already noted the park bench – car park – hiding-under-the-stairs options of the venue, all decision-making requirements and all anticipatory anxiety relating to all of the above. Sorted. I ate this meal sometimes ten times a week for lunches and dinners to avoid ever having to do more than necessary to get food. I stripped the shelves of sardines (boneless and skinless only) and my one preferred flavour of couscous (Moroccan, if you're interested), appearing to all supermarket cashiers as if I had a very well-fed cat. This small step of taking my own food wherever I went was critical to me managing my spoons at times when spoons were in critical supply.

Many of the approaches and strategies used by autistic females to minimize the negative impacts of being autistic in a non-autistic world are either self-generated or developed with the help of the autistic community, which in the case of autistic burnout was years ahead of the research that now exists on the subject. Niamh Garvey's excellent book *Taking Care of Your Autistic Self* (Garvey, 2023) is highly recommended for its wealth of practical information and useful ideas for managing the non-autistic world. Niamh is autistic herself, diagnosed in adulthood as a result of her daughter's diagnosis. Niamh's book takes us step by step through the process of recognizing autistic triggers, 'rationing' them and developing plans from recovery and calming. She also talks us through developing routines and using intense interests to build well-being alongside identifying individual sensory and other triggers, and strategies to minimize their negative impact.

Techniques for managing autistic burnout follow the same lines where self-awareness and energy management can help to prevent the escalation of overwhelm into something more harmful (Mantzalas *et al.*, 2022). Talking to other autistic women (often through online communities) and sharing strategies can reduce the sense of isolation or failure than can result in wondering 'what's wrong with me that I can't function as others do?'

Flo Neville, an autistic postgraduate researcher focusing on autistic well-being, is currently studying the importance of alone-time for autistic people. Many autistic people need frequent time alone to recover from or protect against high levels of sensory and social overwhelm. Sometimes they might need to retreat to a 'sanctuary space' where they feel protected from uncomfortable sensory input and where they do not need to engage with other people. These spaces can be 'cosy', 'interesting' and/or 'set up for preferred activities' (Neville, 2022). Sometimes they might need to 'recharge their batteries' through activities such as reading, gaming, being creative or being out and about in nature. Being 'immersed' in activities helps this recharging process, with some participants describing a 'flow-state' when fully engaged in activities that they love.

Flo has found that lots of standard well-being advice isn't always helpful for autistic people, and her research with late-diagnosed autistic women showed that they found it much easier to care for themselves once they knew they were autistic. They knew that their day-to-day experiences were different, and so they understood that their well-being needs were different too. Autistic women often need to find and develop their own well-being strategies, such as spending time alone, being creative, immersing themselves in their interests, being in nature, stimming and/or finding communities of other neurodivergent people. You can read about some of the health and well-being strategies other autistic people use on the site that Flo runs as part of a team of autistic women.[1]

Therapy is another possible strategy for dealing with the emotions of living in the non-autistic world and for finding strategies to improve the experience. Many women report years spent with often numerous therapists who, while useful in finding ways to manage anxiety or low mood, don't seem to alter the fundamental nature of the person as they had hoped. Some women bounced from one therapist to another, feeling that if only they could find the right one, they would be 'fixed/normal'. I have sought the support of several therapists throughout the years with mostly poor results. I was once told by a hypnotherapist that he wished he had my problems, because I complained of severe anxiety and yet could afford to only work part time (he was holding down two jobs). I gave autism training to another therapist in order to tell him how he should deal with me and show that I wasn't being resistant, but that certain techniques involving imagination were just not going to work for me – I paid for the sessions in which I instructed him – only for him to tell me to 'get over' the unacceptable (to me) behaviour of someone close to me that had led me to near psychosis and that 'everyone behaves like that'. The only positive experiences I have

1 www.AutismHWB.com

had have been with a very no-nonsense life coach who knew nothing about autism and an extremely gentle, spiritual, much older therapist (I ignored the fluffy bits she said that I didn't understand but pretended I did) who I saw before I knew anything about being autistic. She was just so kind to me and helped me to get out of an awfully abusive relationship by helping me see that I didn't have to believe what I was being told by my partner.

> In my late teen years and early 20s, basic talk therapy did not seem to be as helpful since I did not seem to have the insight (regarding my feelings and the feelings of others) necessary to benefit from therapy, and my therapist did not recognize my autism (I was not diagnosed at that time). He seemed puzzled by me and did not seem to know how to help me.

Therapy received mixed reviews amongst those who contributed to this book, with some finding it very helpful and others less so. Those who described positive support appeared to have received input that was directive and supported the learning of social understanding, rather than a more psychoanalytical, emotional 'talking' approach. An understanding of autism as both a starting point and an end goal is crucial when considering any therapeutic support. This allows the therapy to be focused on achieving an autistic quality of life, rather than trying to 'fix' or normalize the autistic woman. Typical therapy may encourage more socializing, variety and new experiences, all of which may be entirely the opposite of what she requires. The result of this, as some women have reported, is that they begin therapy because they feel that they are failing at life, and then feel like they are failing at therapy too by being unable to 'go out and make more friends'. Fortunately, the number of neurodiverse therapists has increased markedly over the past few years, which is a huge relief.

> My current therapist has been the most helpful to me since she understands my autism condition fairly well, and she understands the need to help me with interpreting various social

> situations. She also has gotten me involved in music activities with others, including jamming with other musicians on a weekly basis... She has also gotten me involved in meditation... These activities have also helped me to recognize and see that I am a worthy person with many strengths and perhaps even gifts (so to speak).

> Some counsellors have been useless with me, asking me about my feelings, but my current one has a thorough understanding of AS [Asperger syndrome] and doesn't ask me about my feelings unless I bring them up, which is much better... I need other people to be understanding and not get annoyed with me. I need my partner to put up with being shouted at when he doesn't really deserve it.

Steph Jones' book *The Autistic Survival Guide to Therapy* (forthcoming) is a must-read for any autistic women who has had therapy or is considering it, as well as all therapists whether they have knowingly worked with an autistic person or not. Steph explains how different types of therapy 'fit' with the autistic brain and offers guidance for therapists and strategies for living a good autistic life.

> For me our key task in therapy, coaching or whatever approach feels right is to go back to basics and create a neurodivergent-friendly life which works for us. If you go to therapy essentially asking how to keep up with the neurotypical human experience, you're essentially asking how to hack autism. Can't be done. Sorry. But does an autistic person need psychological therapy because they're autistic? Absolutely not. There is nothing wrong with you. You might need to do some work to adjust your own negative perceptions of yourself after a lifetime of feeling mad, bad and defective, but trust me, you're ace. (Jones, forthcoming, p.215-216)

For the most part (perhaps due to a lack of confidence in clinicians), autistic women find ways to manage their own well-being as best they can in the circumstances. Their awareness of their autism and its negative impact on their health and well-being is key to them being able to develop practical strategies for themselves. For me, the outdoors solves everything. For others it is TV, crafts, cats, sleep or Victorian corsets. Who cares? No one is judging, just find what it is and do more of it.

> Often, I find that the only way to relieve disturbing thoughts or fixations is to engage in positive fixations such as...my music, photography and art videos.

> Exercise has been a great daily activity to ward off stress and tension.

> [...] Time and someone being kind and understanding when I can't cope or become overwhelmed.

> [...] Company, but understanding company.

> [...] My own therapy of writing stuff down, like encouraging thoughts, plans, notes on how to deal with people who upset me, etc.

> I try to keep fit and have taken up roller skating. Walking helps with my depression a great deal.

> I am very driven to create or indulge in creative activities where I can express myself, and I have found such activities and therapy to be vital for my mental health. Without such, I tend to engage in very negative, self-condemning thoughts and sometimes suicidal ideation when depressed. I now recognize the triggers, and I try as much as possible to avoid them and do my best to engage in positive activities and to maintain my commitments to others. I work very hard at trying to improve myself and maintain my well-being.

These girls and women need opportunities to speak to each other and find their own tribe, their own community. This is a place where they can share their trials and tribulations and not get the response, 'You did what?', but instead hear, 'Yeah, I do that too'. This can make all the difference between self-esteem and self-destruction. Local female support groups, online communities and anywhere that autistic girls and women gather are places that they can find their 'home'.

GPs and clinicians are the gatekeepers to a much greater quality of life for these girls and women. These professionals need to learn what to ask, listen to them, look for the autism beneath the facade and believe what they say; and yes, they are 'looking for a label', because that's what opens the door to the right support and knowledge.

Education professionals, support workers and families need to recognize that it may be more than just 'teenage girl stuff', 'neurotic' (that was how I was described) or 'shyness'. It may be something else. Just because she's quiet and not causing you any trouble, don't overlook her. She's not like other girls: don't judge her unfavourably against yourself (as a woman) or other girls/women. She thinks differently; keep an open mind.

Girls and autistic women: please know that you're fine exactly as you are. Yes, you're a bit weird, but that's perfectly alright. You might not feel much like a typical 'woman', but that's okay too – most of us don't. And you're totally right about handbags. You only need one, and that's a rucksack. Don't believe anyone when they say that they want the complete and honest truth; they don't, and they will get upset with you if you tell it to them. Please don't ever, *ever* compare yourself to a neurotypical (NT) girl or woman. They are a different species, and you'll only feel inadequate and bad about yourself because you will compare yourself to them socially, rather than in any of the numerous ways that your ability exceeds theirs. Find your tribe – online, in knitting groups, gaming communities, at comic conventions. Find people who are delighted that you are you. And you should be delighted because you will soon realize (if you haven't already) that all those things you worried about don't matter at all and that there are so many interesting things to get completely engrossed in one at a time. And don't feel bad about changing interests either. Just think of all the amazing stuff that you know how to do.

I hope that this updated version of my book has either given you something new to consider in the world of autistic females, or simply reinforced what you already knew to be so. There are so many things that I will have missed; research, articles, books, blogs, podcasts and videos appear on a daily basis now on the subject of autistic girls and women. Go find them. Connect with others who are on the road with you and maybe further along, or if you don't want to connect with anyone, just lurk on the sidelines and learn from them quietly.

So, for me, after many years of not heeding my own advice by living a very non-autism-compatible life of constant change, lots of people and daily difficult environments, gradually falling apart mentally and physically through a likely combination of autistic burnout and a lengthy and ongoing perimenopause, I gave it all up. Now, by necessity, I live in a manner that I hope all autistic women have the opportunity to live in – *before* it becomes a necessity. My life is very small. I cannot travel alone. I work part time from home to pay the bills because that is all I can manage (even then with anxiety, naps and headaches). I spend my time mostly outdoors making and growing things, because that is what brings me joy and means I don't hurt. A typical life doesn't work for me, and I give myself permission to not feel bad about that. And so can you.

Unconventional people need unconventional solutions. I hope that you are all able to find yours, or those for the autistic girls and women in your life and in your care. Look after yourselves (and them). You're alright just as you are.

References

American Psychiatric Association (2013) *Diagnostic and statistical manual of mental disorders, fifth edition, DSM-5*. Arlington, VA: American Psychiatric Association.

Attwood, T. (2007) *Complete guide to Asperger's Syndrome*. London: Jessica Kingsley Publishers.

Attwood, T. (2012) 'Girls with Asperger's Syndrome: early diagnosis is critical', *Autism Asperger's Digest*, July/August. Available at www.autismdigest.com/girls-with-a (Accessed: 22 November 2014).

Attwood, T. (2013) 'Girls' Questionnaire for Autism Spectrum Conditions (GQ-ASC)'. For more details, visit Professor Attwood's website at www.tonyattwood.com.au.

Attwood, T. *et al.* (2006) *Asperger's and Girls*. Arlington, TX: Future Horizons.

Autism Women Matter (2013) 'Autism Women Matter Survey, 2013. Available at www.autismwomenmatter.org.uk/survey (Accessed: 22 November 2014).

Auyeung, B. *et al.* (2009) 'Fetal testosterone and autistic traits', *British Psychological Society*, 100(Pt 1), pp.1–22. doi: 10.1348/000712608X311731

Babb, C. *et al.* (2021) '"It's not that they don't want to access the support . . . it's the impact of the autism": the experience of eating disorder services from the perspective of autistic women, parents and healthcare professionals', *Autism*, 25(5), pp.1409–1421. doi: 10.1177/1362361321991257

Backer van Ommeren, T. *et al.* (2016) 'Sex difference in the reciprocal behaviour of children with autism', *Autism*, 21(6), pp.795–803. doi: 10.1177/1362361316669622

Baeza-Velasco, C. *et al.* (2018) 'Autism, Joint Hypermobility-Related Disorders and Pain'. *Frontiers in Psychiatry*, 9(656). doi: 10.3389/fpsyt.2018.00656

Baldwin, S. and Costley, D. (2016) 'The experiences and needs of female adults with high-functioning autism spectrum disorder', *Autism*, 20(4), pp.483–495. doi: 10.3389/fpsyt.2018.00656

Bargiela, S. *et al.* (2016) 'The experiences of late-diagnosed women with autism spectrum conditions: an investigation of the female autism phenotype', *Journal of Autism and Development Disorders*, 46(10), pp.3281–3294. doi: 10.1007/s10803-016-2872-8

Baron-Cohen, S. (2002) 'The extreme male brain theory of autism', *Trends in Cognitive Science*, 6(6), pp.248–254. doi: 10.1016/s1364-6613(02)01904-6

Baron-Cohen, S. and Wheelwright, S. (2003) 'The Friendship Questionnaire: an investigation of adults with Asperger syndrome or high-functioning autism and normal sex differences', *Journal of Autism and Developmental Disorders*, 33(3), pp.509–517. doi: 10.1023/a:1025879411971

Baron-Cohen, S. *et al.* (2013) 'Do girls with anorexia nervosa have elevated autistic traits?', *Molecular Autism*, 4(24). doi: org/10.1186/2040-2392-4-24

Beardon, L. (2017) *Autism and Asperger syndrome in adults.* London: Sheldon Press.

Bejerot, S. *et al.* (2012) 'The extreme male brain revisited: gender coherence in adults with autism spectrum disorder', *British Journal of Psychiatry*, 201(2), pp.116–123. doi: 10.1192/bjp.bp.111.09789

Bölte, S. *et al.* (2011) 'Sex differences in cognitive domains and their clinical correlates in higher-functioning autism spectrum disorders', *Autism*, 15(4), pp.497–511. doi: 10.1177/1362361310391116

Brown, C.M. *et al.* (2020) 'Am I autistic? Utility of the Girls Questionnaire for Autism Spectrum Condition as an autism assessment in adult women' *Autism in Adulthood*, 2(3), pp.216–226. doi: 10.1089/aut.2019.0054

Buchan, L. (2022) Personal communication, 17 October 2022.

Burke, L.M. *et al.* (2010) 'Gynecologic issues with Down syndrome, autism, and cerebral palsy', *Journal of Pediatric and Adolescent Gynecology*, 23(1), pp.11–15. doi: 10.1016/j.jpag.2009.04.005

Burkett, C. (2020) '"Autistic while black": how autism amplifies stereotypes'. Available at www.spectrumnews.org/opinion/viewpoint/autistic-while-black-how-autism-amplifies-stereotypes/ (Accessed: 24 May 2023).

Bursch, B. *et al.* (2004) 'Chronic pain in individuals with previously undiagnosed autistic spectrum disorders', *Journal of Pain*, 5(5), pp.290–295. doi: 10.1016/j.jpain.2004.04.004

Carter, A.S. *et al.* (2007) 'Sex differences in toddlers with autism spectrum disorders', *Journal of Autism and Developmental Disorders*, 37(1), pp.86–97. doi: 10.1007/s10803-006-0331-7

Casanova, E.L. *et al.* (2020) 'The relationship between autism and Ehlers–Danlos syndromes/hypermobility spectrum disorders', *Journal of Personalized Medicine*, 10(4), p.260. doi: 10.3390/jpm10040260

Cassidy, S. *et al.* (2014) 'Suicidal ideation and suicide plans or attempts in adults with Asperger's syndrome attending a specialist diagnostic clinic: a clinical cohort study', *The Lancet Psychiatry*, 1(2), pp.142–147. doi: 10.1016/S2215-0366(14)70248-2

Cassidy, S.A. *et al.* (2020) 'Is camouflaging autistic traits associated with suicidal thoughts and behaviours? Expanding the interpersonal psychological theory of suicide in an undergraduate student sample', *Journal of Autism and Developmental Disorders*, 50(10), pp.3638–3648. doi: 10.1007/s10803-019-04323-3

Cazalis, F. *et al.* (2022) 'Evidence that nine autistic women out of ten have been victims of sexual violence', *Frontiers in Behavioral Neuroscience*, 16, p.852203. doi: 10.3389/fnbeh.2022.852203

Charlton, R. (2017) 'Researching autism and ageing'. National Autistic Society. Available at www.autism.org.uk/advice-and-guidance/professional-practice/research-ageing. (Accessed: 24 May 2023.)

Chellew, T. *et al.* (2022) 'The early childhood signs of autism in females: a systematic review', *Review Journal of Autism and Developmental Disorders*. doi: 10.1007/s40489-022-00337-3

Cherskov, A. *et al.* (2018) 'Polycystic ovary syndrome and autism: a test of the prenatal sex steroid theory', *Translational Psychiatry*, 8(1), p.136. doi: 10.1038/s41398-018-0186-7

Craig, M.C. *et al.* (2007) 'Women with autistic-spectrum disorder: magnetic resonance imaging study of brain anatomy', *British Journal of Psychiatry*, 191(3), pp.224–228. doi: 10.1192/bjp.bp.106.034603

Cridland, L. *et al.* (2014) 'Being a girl in a boys' world: investigating the experiences of girls with autism spectrum disorders during adolescence', *Journal of Autism and Developmental Disorders*, 44(6), pp.1261–1274. doi: 10.1007/s10803-013-1985-6

Cumin, J. *et al.* (2022) 'Positive and differential diagnosis of autism in verbal women of typical intelligence: a Delphi study', *Autism*, 26(5), pp.1153–1164. doi: 10.1177/13623613211042719

D'Mello, A.M. *et al.* (2022) 'Exclusion of females in autism research: empirical evidence for a "leaky" recruitment-to-research pipeline', *Autism Research*, 15(10), pp.1929–1940. doi.org/10.1002/aur.2795

de Vries, A.L. *et al.* (2010) 'Autism spectrum disorders in gender dysphoric children and adolescents', *Journal of Autism and Developmental Disorders*, 40(8), pp.930–936. doi: 10.1007/s10803-010-0935-9

Dewinter, J. *et al.* (2017) 'Sexual orientation, gender identity, and romantic relationships in adolescents and adults with autism spectrum disorder', *Journal of Autism and Developmental Disorders*, 47(9), pp.2927–2934. doi: 10.1007/s10803-017-3199-9

Diemer, C.D. *et al.* (2022) 'Autism presentation in female and Black populations: examining the roles of identity, theory, and systemic inequalities', *Autism*, 26(8), pp.1931–1946. doi: 10.1177/13623613221113501

Dugdale, A.-S. *et al.* (2021) 'Intense connection and love: the experiences of autistic mothers', *Autism*, 25(7), pp.1973–1984. doi: 10.1177/13623613211005987

Eaton, L. (2012) 'Under the radar and behind the scenes: the perspectives of mothers with daughters on the autism spectrum', *Good Autism Practice*, 13(2), pp.9–17.

Frazier, T.W. *et al.* (2014) 'Behavioral and cognitive characteristics of females and autistic males in the Simons Simplex Collection', *Journal of the American Academy of Child and Adolescent Psychiatry*, 53(3), pp.329–340. doi: 10.1016/j.jaac.2013.12.004

Freeman, N.C. and Grigoriadis, A. (2023) 'A survey of assessment practices among health professionals diagnosing females with autism', *Research in Developmental Disabilities*, 135,104445. doi: 10.1016/j.ridd.2023.104445

Full Spectrum Child Care (2020) 'The forgotten girls: racial and ethnic disparities within the disability community through the lenses of Black women and girls with autism'. Available at www.fullspectrumchildcare.com/blog/the-forgotten-girls-racial-and-ethnic-disparities-within-the-disability-community-through-the-lenses-of-black-women-and-girls-with-autism (Accessed: 24 May 2023).

Garvey, N. (2023) *Looking after your autistic self: a personalized self-care approach to managing your sensory and emotional wellbeing.* London: Jessica Kingsley Publishers.

Gaus, V. (2007) *Cognitive behavioural therapy for adult Asperger syndrome.* New York, NY: Guilford Press.

Gaus, V. (2011) *Living well on the spectrum.* New York, NY: The Guilford Press.

Giarelli, E. *et al.* (2010) 'Sex differences in the evaluation and diagnosis of autism spectrum disorders among children', *Disability and Health Journal*, 3(2), pp.107–116. doi: 10.1016/j.dhjo.2009.07.001

Gillberg, C. (1983) 'Are autism and anorexia nervosa related?', *British Journal of Psychiatry*, 142(4), p.428. doi: 10.1192/bjp.142.4.428b

Gilmour, L. *et al.* (2012) 'Sexuality in a community based sample of autistic adults spectrum disorder', *Research in Autism Spectrum Disorders*, 6(1), pp.313–318. doi: 10.1016/j.rasd.2011.06.003

Glans, M.R. *et al.* (2022) 'The relationship between generalised joint hypermobility and autism spectrum disorder in adults: a large, cross-sectional, case control comparison', *Frontiers in Psychiatry*, 12, 803334. doi: 10.3389/fpsyt.2021.803334

Glidden, D. *et al.* (2015) 'Gender dysphoria and autism spectrum disorder: a systemic review of the literature', *Sexual Medicine Reviews*, 4(1), pp.3–14. doi: 10.1016/j.sxmr.2015.10.003

Goodwin, D.W. (1988) *Alcohol and the writer.* London: Penguin Books.

Gould, J. (2014) Personal communication, 10 January 2014.

Gould, J. and Ashton-Smith, J. (2011) 'Missed diagnosis or misdiagnosis? Girls and women on the autism spectrum', *Good Autism Practice*, 12(1), pp.34–41.

Grant, A. *et al.* (2022) 'Autistic women's view and experiences of infant feeding: a systematic review of qualitative evidence', *Autism*, 26(6), pp.1341–1352. doi: 10.1177/13623613221089374

Griffin, C. *et al.* (2016) 'Alexithymia in children with and without autism spectrum disorders', *Autism Research*, 9(7), pp.773–780. doi: 10.1002/aur.1569

Hamilton, A. *et al.* (2011) 'Autism spectrum disorders and menstruation', *Journal of Adolescent Health*, 49(4), pp.443–445. doi: 10.1016/j.jadohealth.2011.01.015

Happé, F. and Charlton, R.A. (2012) 'Aging in autism spectrum disorders: a mini-review', *Gerontology*, 58(1), pp.70–78. doi: 10.1159/000329720

Hartley, S.L. and Sikora, D.M. (2009) 'Sex differences in autism spectrum disorder: an examination of developmental functioning, autistic symptoms, and coexisting behaviour problems in toddlers', *Journal of Autism and Developmental Disorders*, 39(12), pp.1715–1722. doi: 10.1007/s10803-009-0810-8

Head, A.M. *et al.* M.A. (2014) 'Gender differences in emotionality and sociability in children with autistic spectrum disorders', *Molecular Autism*, 5(1), p.19. doi: 10.1186/2040-2392-5-19

Hendrickx, S. (2008) *Love, sex and long-term relationships: what people with Asperger Syndrome really really want.* London: Jessica Kingsley Publishers.

Hendrickx, S. (2009) *Asperger Syndrome and employment: what people with Asperger Syndrome really really want.* London: Jessica Kingsley Publishers.

Hendrickx, S. and Newton, K. (2007) *Asperger Syndrome – a love story.* London: Jessica Kingsley Publishers.

Heylens, G. *et al.* (2018) 'The co-occurrence of gender dysphoria and autism spectrum disorder in adults: an analysis of cross-sectional and clinical chart data', *Journal of Autism and Developmental Disorders*, 48(6), pp.2217–2223. doi: 10.1007/s10803-018-3480-6

Higgins, J.M. *et al.* (2021) 'Defining autistic burnout through experts by lived experience: Grounded Delphi method investigation #AutisticBurnout', *Autism*, 25(8), pp.2356–2369. doi: 10.1177/13623613211019858

Hirvikoski, T. *et al.* (2020) 'Individual risk and familial liability for suicide attempt and suicide in autism: a population-based study', *Psychological Medicine*, 50(9), pp.1463–1474. doi: 10.1017/S0033291719001405

Hisle-Gorman, E. *et al.* (2019) 'Gender dysphoria in children with autism spectrum disorder', *LGBT Health*, 6(3), pp. 95–100. doi: 10.1089/lgbt.2018.0252

Holliday Willey, L. (2001) *Asperger Syndrome in the family.* London: Jessica Kingsley Publishers.

Holliday Willey, L. (2012) *Safety skills for Asperger women: how to save a perfectly good female life.* London: Jessica Kingsley Publishers.

Holliday Willey, L. (2014) *Pretending to be normal: living with Asperger's syndrome.* London: Jessica Kingsley Publishers.

Hull, L. *et al.* (2020) 'The female autism phenotype and camouflaging: a narrative review', *Review Journal of Autism and Developmental Disorders*, 7(4), pp.306–317. doi: 10.1007/s40489-020-00197-9

Hurley, E. (ed.) (2014) *Ultraviolet voices: stories of women on the autism spectrum.* Birmingham: Autism West Midlands.

Hwang, Y.I. *et al.* (2020) 'Aging well on the autism spectrum: an examination of the dominant model of successful aging', *Journal of Autism and Developmental Disorders*, 50(7), pp.2326–2335. doi: 10.1007/s10803-018-3596-8

Impact Initiatives, Asperger's Voice Self-Advocacy Group & West Sussex Asperger Awareness Group (2013) *Mental health services for adults with Asperger's syndrome and HFA in West Sussex: a quality check.* Littlehampton: Impact Initiatives.

Ingudomnukul, E. *et al.* (2007) 'Elevated rates of testosterone-related disorders in women with autistic spectrum conditions', *Hormones and Behavior*, 51(5), pp.597–604. doi: 10.1016/j.yhbeh.2007.02.001

Jacquemont, S. *et al.* (2014) 'A higher mutational burden in females supports a "female protective model" in neurodevelopmental disorders', *American Journal of Human Genetics*, 94(3), pp.415–425. doi: 10.1016/j.ajhg.2014.02.001

Jansen, H. and Rombout, B. (2014) *Autipower: successful living and working with an autism spectrum disorder.* London: Jessica Kingsley Publishers.

Jones, S. (2023) Personal communication, 2023.

Jones, S. (forthcoming) *The autistic survival guide to therapy.* London: Jessica Kingsley Publishers.

Kallitsounaki, A. *et al.* (2021) 'Links between autistic traits, feelings of gender dysphoria, and mentalising ability: replication and extension of previous findings from the general population', *Journal of Autism and Developmental Disorders*, 51(5), pp.1458–1465. doi: 10.1007/s10803-020-04626-w

Kanner, L. (1943) 'Autistic disturbances of affective contact', *Nervous Child*, 2, pp.217–250.

Karavidas, M. and de Visser, R.O. (2022) '"It's not just in my head, and it's not just irrelevant": autistic negotiations of menopausal transitions', *Journal of Autism and Developmental Disorders*, 52(3), pp.1143–1155. doi: 10.1007/s10803-021-05010-y

Kavanaugh, B. *et al.* (2023) 'Moderators of age of diagnosis in > 20,000 females with autism in two large US studies', *Journal of Autism and Developmental Disorders*, 53(2), pp.864–869. doi: 10.1007/s10803-021-05026-4

Kearns Miller, J. (2003) *Women from another planet?* Bloomington, IN: 1st Books Library.

Kim, C. (2014) *Nerdy, shy and socially inappropriate: a user guide to an Asperger life.* London: Jessica Kingsley Publishers.

Knickmeyer, R.C. *et al.* (2008) 'Sex-typical play: masculinization/defeminization in girls with an autism spectrum condition' *Journal of Autism and Developmental Disorders*, 38(6), pp.1028–1035. doi: 10.1007/s10803-007-0475-0

Kock, E. *et al.* (2019) 'Autistic women's experience of intimate relationships: the impact of an adult diagnosis', *Advances in Autism*, 5(1), pp.38–49. doi: 10.1108/AIA-09-2018-0035

Kopp, S. and Gillberg, C. (1992) 'Girls with social deficits and learning problems: autism, atypical Asperger syndrome or a variant of these conditions', *European Child and Adolescent Psychiatry*, 1(2), pp.89–99. doi: 10.1007/BF02091791

Kopp, S. and Gillberg, C. (2011) 'The Autism Spectrum Screening Questionnaire (ASSQ)-Revised Extended Version (ASSQ-REV): an instrument for better capturing the autism phenotype in girls? A preliminary study involving 191 clinical cases and community controls', *Research in Developmental Disabilities*, 32(6), pp.2875–2888. doi: 10.1016/j.ridd.2011.05.017

Kosidou, K. *et al.* (2016) 'Maternal polycystic ovary syndrome and the risk of autism spectrum disorders in the offspring: a population-based nationwide study in Sweden', *Molecular Psychiatry*, 21(10), pp.1441–1448. doi: 10.1038/mp.2015.183

Kotowicz, A. (2022) *What I mean when I say I'm autistic.* Rockville, MD: Neurobeautiful.

Kreiser, N.L. and White, S.W. (2014) 'ASD in females: are we overstating the gender difference in diagnosis?', *Clinical Child and Family Psychology Review*, 17(1), pp.67–84. doi: 10.1007/s10567-013-0148-9

Lai, M.-C. *et al.* (2011) 'A behavioral comparison of male and female adults with high functioning autism spectrum conditions', *PLOS One*, 6(6), e20835. doi: 10.1371/journal.pone.0020835

Lai, M.-C. *et al.* (2013) 'Biological sex affects the neurobiology of autism', *Brain*, 136(9), pp.2799–2815. doi: 10.1093/brain/awt216

Lai, M.-C. *et al.* (2019) 'Neural self representation in autistic women and association with "compensatory camouflaging"', *Autism*, 23(5), pp.1210–1223. doi: 10.1177/1362361318807159

Lawson, W. (2000) *Life behind glass: a personal account of autism spectrum disorder.* London: Jessica Kingsley Publishers.

Lawson, W. (2014) Personal communication, 9 October 2014.

Lee, D.O. (2004) 'Menstrually related self-injurious behavior in adolescents with autism', *Journal of the American Academy of Child and Adolescent Psychiatry*, 43(10), p.1193. doi: 10.1097/01.chi.0000135624.89971.d1

Lemon, J.M. *et al.* (2011) 'Executive functioning in autism spectrum disorders: a gender comparison of response inhibition', *Journal of Autism and Developmental Disorders*, 41(3), pp.352–356. doi: 10.1007/s10803-010-1039-2

Linden, W. *et al.* (1995) 'Measuring alexithymia: reliabilty, validity, and prevalence', in J. Butcher and C. Speilberger (eds). *Advances in personality assessment.* Mahwah, NJ: Lawrence Erlbaum, pp.51–95.

Livingston, L.A. and Happé, F. (2017) 'Conceptualising compensation in neurodevelopmental disorders: reflections from autism spectrum disorder', *Neuroscience and Biobehavioral Reviews*, 80, pp.729–742. doi: 10.1016/j.neubiorev.2017.06.005

Loomes, R. *et al.* (2017) 'What is the male-to-female ratio in autism spectrum disorder? A systematic review and meta-analysis', *Journal of American Academy of Child and Adolescent Psychiatry*, 56(6), pp.466–474. doi: 10.1016/j.jaac.2017.03.013

Lord, C. *et al.* (1982) 'Sex differences in autism', *Journal of Autism and Developmental Disorders*, 12(4), pp.317–330. doi: 10.1007/BF01538320

Mandy, W. (2013) 'DSM-5 may better serve autistic girls'. New York: Simons Foundation Autism Research Initiative. Available at www.sfari.org/news-and-opinion/specials/2013/dsm-5-special-report/dsm-5-may-better-serve-girls-with-autism (Accessed: 24 May 2023).

Mandy, W. *et al.* (2012) 'Sex differences in autism spectrum disorder: evidence from a large sample of children and adolescents', *Journal of Autism and Developmental Disorders*, 42(7), pp.1304–1313. doi: 10.1007/s10803-011-1356-0

Mantzalas, J. *et al.* (2022) 'What is autistic burnout? A thematic analysis of posts on two online platforms', *Autism in Adulthood*, 4(1), pp.52–65. doi: 10.1089/aut.2021.0021

Martini, M.I. *et al.* (2022) 'Sex differences in mental health problems and psychiatric hospitalization in autistic young adults', *JAMA Psychiatry*, 79(12), pp.1188–1198. doi: 10.1001/jamapsychiatry.2022.3475

McCarthy, M.M. *et al.* (2012) 'Sex differences in the brain: the not so inconvenient truth'. *Journal of Neuroscience*, 32(7), pp.2241–2247. doi: 10.1523/JNEUROSCI.5372-11.2012

McLennan, J.D. *et al.* (1993) 'Sex differences in higher functioning autistic people', *Journal of Autism and Developmental Disorders*, 23(2), pp.217–227. doi: 10.1007/BF01046216

Michael, C. (2015) 'Autism, ageing and women: not invisible, just ignored'. National Autistic Society. Available at https://www.autism.org.uk/advice-and-guidance/professional-practice/women-ageing/ (Accessed: 24 May 2023).

Milner, V. *et al.* (2019) 'A qualitative exploration of the female experience of autism spectrum disorder (ASD)', *Journal of Autism and Developmental Disorders*, 49(6), pp.2389–2402. doi: 10.1007/s10803-019-03906-4

Miserandino, C. (2003) 'The spoon theory'. Available at https://butyoudontlooksick.com/articles/written-by-christine/the-spoon-theory/ (Accessed: 24 May 2023).

Moreno, S.J. (2018) 'Autism after 65: making the most of the golden years'. Indiana Resource Center for Autism, Indiana University Bloomington. Available at www.iidc.indiana.edu/irca/articles/autism-after-65.html (Accessed: 24 May 2023).

Moseley, R.L. *et al.* (2020) '"When my autism broke": a qualitative study spotlighting autistic voices on menopause', *Autism*, 24(6), pp.1423–1437. doi: 10.1177/1362361319901184

Moseley, R.L. *et al.* (2021) 'Autism research is "all about the blokes and the kids": autistic women breaking the silence on menopause', *British Journal of Health Psychology*, 26, pp.709–726. doi: 10.1111/bjhp.12477

National Autistic Society (2013a) 'Autism and ageing: older people's stories'. Available at www.autism.org.uk/living-with-autism/adults-with-autism-or-asperger-syndrome/autism-and-ageing/older-peoples-stories.aspx (Accessed: 22 November 2014).

National Autistic Society (2013b) *Getting on: growing older with autism – a policy report.* London: National Autistic Society.

National Collaborating Centre for Mental Health (2012) *Autism: the NICE guideline on recognition, referral, diagnosis and management of adults on the autism spectrum.* London: British Psychological Society and Royal College of Psychiatrists.

Neville, F. (2019) 'Autistics, autodidacts and autonomy: exploring how late diagnosed autistic women in the UK and US self-manage their health and wellbeing with dietary and other lifestyle measures'. Dissertation [online]. MRes, University of the West of England. Available at https://florenceneville.com/research-and-writing/ (Accessed: 24 May 2023).

Neville, F. (2022) 'Reacting, retreating, regulating and reconnecting: summary of study findings'. Available at https://autismhwb.com/reacting-retreating-regulating-and-reconnecting (Accessed: 24 May 2023).

Nichols, S. *et al.* (2009) *Girls growing up on the autism spectrum.* London: Jessica Kingsley Publishers.

Nyden, A. *et al.* (2000) 'Autism spectrum and attention deficit disorders in girls: some neuropsychological aspects', *European Child and Adolescent Psychiatry*, 9(3), pp.180–185. doi: 10.1007/s007870070041

Obaydi, H. and Puri, B.K. (2008) 'Prevalence of premenstrual syndrome in autism: a prospective observer-related study', *Journal of International Medical Research*, 36(2), pp.268–272. doi: 10.1177/147323000803600208

Ola, L. and Gullon-Scott, F. (2020) 'Facial emotion recognition in autistic adult females correlates with alexithymia, not autism', *Autism*, 24(8), pp.2021–2034. doi: 10.1177/1362361320932727

Oldershaw, A. *et al.* (2011) 'Is anorexia nervosa a version of autism spectrum disorders?' *European Eating Disorders Review*, 19(6), pp.462–474. doi: 10.1002/erv.1069

Pelz-Sherman, D. (2014) 'Supporting breastfeeding among women on the autistic spectrum', *Clinical Lactation*, 5(2), pp.62–66. doi: 10.1002/erv.1069

Petitpierre, G. *et al.* (2021) 'Eating behaviour in autism: senses as a window towards food acceptance', *Current Opinion in Food Science*, 41, pp.210–216. doi: 10.1016/j.cofs.2021.04.015

Pohl, A. *et al.* (2014) 'Uncovering steroidopathy in autistic women: a latent class analysis', *Molecular Autism*, 5, p.27. doi: 10.1186/2040-2392-5-27

Pohl, A.L. *et al.* (2020) 'A comparative study of autistic and non-autistic women's experience of motherhood', *Molecular Autism*, 11, p.3. doi: 10.1186/s13229-019-0304-2

Poquérusse, J. *et al.* (2018) 'Alexithymia and autism spectrum disorder: a complex relationship', *Frontiers in Psychology*, 9, p.1196. doi: 10.3389/fpsyg.2018.01196

Råstam, M. (2008) 'Eating disturbances in autism spectrum disorders with focus on adolescent and adult years', *Clinical Neuropsychiatry: Journal of Treatment Evaluation*, 5(1), pp.31–42. https://psycnet.apa.org/record/2008-07906-005

Ratto, A.B. *et al.* (2022) 'Centering the inner experience of autism: development of the Self-Assessment of Autistic Traits', *Autism in Adulthood*, 5(1), pp.93–105. doi: 10.1089/aut.2021.0099

Raymaker, D.M. *et al.* (2020) 'Having all of your internal resources exhausted beyond measure and being left with no clean-up crew: defining autistic burnout', *Autism in Adulthood*, 2(2), pp.132–143. doi: 10.1089/aut.2019.0079

Riley-Hall, E. (2012) *Parenting girls on the autism spectrum*. London: Jessica Kingsley Publishers.

Rozsa, M. (2017) 'Black, female and autistic – hiding in plain sight'. Available at www.salon.com/2017/03/15/listen-black-female-and-autistic-hiding-in-plain-sight/ (Accessed: 24 May 2023).

Ruigrok, A.N.V. *et al.* (2014) 'A meta-analysis of sex differences in human brain structure', *Neuroscience & Biobehavioral Reviews*, 39(100), pp.34–50. doi:10.1016/j.neubiorev.2013.12.004

Russell, G. *et al.* (2011) 'Social and demographic factors that influence the diagnosis of autistic spectrum disorders', *Social Psychiatry and Psychiatric Epidemiology*, 46(12), pp.1283–1293. Doi: 10.1007/s00127-010-0294-z

Rynkiewicz, A. *et al.* (2016) 'An investigation of the "female camouflage effect" in autism using a computerized ADOS-2 and a test of sex/gender differences', *Molecular Autism*, 7, 10. doi: 10.1186/s13229-016-0073-0

Schembari, M. (2023) Personal communication, 17 January 2023.

Schembari, M. (forthcoming) *A little less broken*. New York, NY: Flatiron Books.

Schnitzler, E. (2022) 'The neurology and psychopathology of Pica', *Current Neurology and Neuroscience Reports*, 22(8), pp.531–536. doi: 10.1007/s11910-022-01218-2

Schröder, S.S. *et al.* (2022) 'Problematic eating behaviours of autistic women: a scoping review', *European Eating Disorders Review*, 30(5), pp.510–537. doi: 10.1002/erv.2932

Sedgewick, F. (2018) 'Examining the peer relationships and conflict experiences of adolescent girls and women on the autism spectrum'. PhD thesis, University College London Institute of Education.

Shea, L. *et al.* (2019) 'Understanding and managing Pica'. Available at www.autism.org.uk/advice-and-guidance/professional-practice/managing-pica (Accessed: 24 May 2023).

Simone, R. (2010) *Aspergirls*. London: Jessica Kingsley Publishers.

Steinbeck, J. (2001/1962) *Travels with Charley: in search of America*. London: Penguin.

Steward, R. *et al.* (2018) '"Life is much more difficult to manage during periods": autistic experiences of menstruation', *Journal of Autism and Developmental Disorders*, 48(12), pp.4287–4292. doi: 10.1007/s10803-018-3664-0

Stewart, C. (2012) '"Where can we be what we are?": the experiences of girls with Asperger syndrome and their mothers', *Good Autism Practice*, 13(1), pp.40–48.

Stewart, C. (2022) Personal communication, 31 October 2022.

Tchanturia, K. (2021) *Supporting autistic people with eating disorders: a guide to adapting treatment and supporting recovery*. London: Jessica Kingsley Publishers.

Tchanturia, K. *et al.* (2013) 'Exploring autistic traits in anorexia: a clinical study', *Molecular Autism*, 4(1), p.44. doi: 10.1186/2040-2392-4-44

Tierney, S. *et al.* (2016) 'Looking behind the mask: social coping strategies of girls on the autistic spectrum', *Research in Autism Spectrum Disorders*, 23, pp.73–83. doi: 10.1016/j.rasd.2015.11.013

Tinsley, M. and Hendrickx, S. (2008) *Asperger syndrome and alcohol: drinking to cope.* London: Jessica Kingsley Publishers.

Torenvliet, C. *et al.* (2023) 'A longitudinal study on cognitive aging in autism'. *Psychiatry Research*, 321, 115063. doi: 10.1016/j.psychres.2023.115063

Tsai, L.Y. and Beisler, J.M. (1983) 'The development of sex differences in infantile autism', *British Journal of Psychiatry*, 142, pp.373–378. doi: 10.1192/bjp.142.4.373

van der Miesen, A.I.R. *et al.* (2016) 'Gender dysphoria and autism spectrum disorder: a narrative review' *International Review of Psychiatry*, 28(1), pp.70–80. doi: 10.3109/09540261.2015.1111199

van der Miesen, A. *et al.* (2018) 'Prevalence of the wish to be of the opposite gender in adolescents and adults with autism spectrum disorder', *Archives of Sexual Behaviour*, 47(8), pp.2307–2317. doi: 10.1007/s10508-018-1218-3

van Wijngaarden-Cremers, P. and van der Gaag, R. (2015) 'Addiction and autism spectrum disorder', in G. Domm and F. Moggi (eds) *Co-occurring addictive and psychiatric disorders: a practice-based handbook from a European perspective.* Berlin: Springer-Verlag.

Volkmar, F.R. *et al.* (1993) 'Sex differences in pervasive developmental disorders', *Journal of Autism and Developmental Disorders*, 23(4), pp.579–591. doi: 10.1007/BF01046103

Wagner, S. (2006) 'Educating the female student with Asperger's', in T. Attwood *et al.* (eds) *Asperger's and Girls.* Arlington, TX: Future Horizons.

Warrier, V. *et al.* (2020) 'Elevated rates of autism, other neurodevelopmental and psychiatric diagnoses, and autistic traits in transgender and gender-diverse individuals', *Nature Communications*, 11(1), 3959. doi: 10.1038/s41467-020-17794-1

West, E.A. *et al.* (2016) 'Racial and ethnic diversity of participants in research supporting evidence-based practices for learners with autism spectrum disorder', *Journal of Special Education*, 50(3). doi: 10.1177/0022466916632495

Wiggins, L.D. *et al.* (2019) 'Disparities in documented diagnoses of autism spectrum disorder based on demographic, individual, and service factors', *Autism Research*, 13(3), pp.464-473. doi: ord/10.1002/aur.2255

Wilson, C.E. *et al.* (2016) 'Does sex influence the diagnostic evaluation of autism spectrum disorder in adults?', *Autism*, 20(7), pp.808–819. doi: 10.1177/1362361315611381

Wing, L. (1981) 'Sex ratios in early childhood autism and related conditions', *Psychiatry Research*, 5(2), pp.129–137. doi: 10.1016/0165-1781(81)90043-3

Wylie, P. (2014) *Very late diagnosis of Asperger syndrome: how seeking a diagnosis in adulthood can change your life.* London: Jessica Kingsley Publishers.

Zahn-Waxler, C. *et al.* (2008) 'Disorders of childhood and adolescence: gender and psychopathology', *Annual Review of Clinical Psychology*, 4, pp.275–303. doi: 10.1146/annurev.clinpsy.3.022806.091358

Subject Index

Author Index